The
Pied Pipers
of Pot

*Protecting Youth
from the Marijuana Industry*

Pamela McColl

with Emma Todd

Library and Archives Canada Cataloguing in Publication

McColl, Pamela, 1958–, author
The pied pipers of pot : protecting youth from the marijuana industry
/ Pamela McColl.

Includes bibliographical references and index.
Issued in print and electronic formats.
ISBN 978-1-927979-14-3 (softcover).—ISBN 978-1-927979-16-7 (HTML).
—ISBN 978-1-927979-17-4 (PDF)

1. Marijuana abuse—Prevention. 2. Marijuana—Risk assessment.
3. Marijuana—Social aspects. 4. Marijuana—Health aspects. I. Title.

HV5822.M3M33 2017   362.29'57   C2017-901173-1
C2017-901174-X

Cover illustration: Pat Brennan

Grafton and Scratch Publishers
www.graftonandscratch.com

Humpty Dumpty sat on a wall,
Humpty Dumpty had a great fall.

All the king's horses and all the king's men
couldn't put Humpty together again.

"The value of the drug debate as a badge of moral and political affiliation is too potent to allow inconvenient truths to intrude. The reality of less use and less harm has to be airbrushed out of the debate if the power of the opposing polemics is to be sustained."[1]

—PAUL HAYES, HON. PROFESSOR, LONDON SCHOOL OF HYGIENE AND TROPICAL MEDICINE

Contents

Introduction

"Spirit Airlines, playing off the approved use and sale of cannabis in the Rocky Mountain State, dangles discounted fares to Colorado where, its ad informs, 'the no smoking sign is off', nudging the content needle inside a sales niche called marijuana marketing."[2] —Bill Briggs (*CNBC*), 2014

The Pied Pipers of Pot—protecting youth from the marijuana industry, is not investigative in nature, but rather relies on information, argument and scientific evidence available on the public record. This publication tracks the normalization of marijuana products and the advance of the North American marijuana industry in recent years. The material was collected over a five year time period that began in 2012.

"It's become one of the great social experiments of our time," said Governor John Hickenlooper of Colorado, in discussions on marijuana legalization with Chuck Todd of *Meet the Press* (*NBC*), on February 26, 2017. The central question raised by *The Pied Pipers of Pot* is whether "experimenting" with marijuana policy is a risk worth taking; especially during the current period of high rates of use by youth. This question has particular relevance as many young people, in Canada and the United States, have taken to high potency, modified marijuana products, that they prefer to experience through smoking. Survey results clearly identify that many young people are vulnerable, as they are either under-educated, ill-informed or dismissive of the evidence from scientific study that correlates marijuana products with harm. The following discussion addresses this problem.

"No one has a visual yet as to who is behind Big Marijuana. So I want them to start coming out of the shadows. You know, I welcome the fact that they're all starting to show up because I want the American people to really know what's motivating this whole industry and what it is, is big money and its greed. This is about a commercial for profit behemoth coming in to prey on your kids, addict them and to make money off of them at your expense."[3] —Patrick J. Kennedy, former United States representative for the State of Rhode Island

The North American populace is experiencing a "relapse phase" in terms of marijuana use, and once again governments, educators, and parents are deliberating how best to respond to a heavy number of young people becoming regular or even daily users.[4] The historical record and the worldwide variations in rates of use establish that individuals do not just fall into using hallucinogenic substances but rather they are pushed into use during periods dominated by permissive societal drug norms, in cultures that avail ease of access, and that are plagued by predatory profiteers.

The reach of the emerging marijuana industry should not be under-estimated in deducing how youth are initiated to marijuana. Youth can be enticed to use "adult-only" marijuana products, just as they have been lured to take up restricted but legal tobacco and alcohol, and subjected to wide-spread normalization of these products. Virtually all regular tobacco smokers report they started using cigarettes before their eighteenth birthday, which is under the legal age of access in all jurisdictions across North American.

A generation of young people in both Canada and the United States are up against an ambitious and aggressive marijuana industry, who have all the marketing expertise money can garner.

In 2016, Monitoring the Future (MTF) reported that 32% of grade 12 students perceived a risk of harm from the regular use of marijuana, marking the lowest level ever recorded by MTF, which began surveying American students on their behaviors and attitudes in 1975.[4] Low levels of perceived risk have often preceded increases in marijuana prevalence.[4] "Publicity around legalizing medical, and in some cases recreational use, may have served to normalize use of marijuana, the most widely used of all illicit substances."[4] —MTF

In 2013, the Canadian Centre on Substance Abuse (CCSA) surveyed Canadian youth on their perceptions of marijuana.[5] Of those surveyed many held a belief that "everyone smokes weed", viewed abstaining from cannabis as abnormal, and perceived positive effects more often than negative effects. They also were shown to perceive that marijuana products had the ability to help a person focus, relax, sleep, be less violent and that marijuana improved creativity, and purified the body.[5] Peer pressure, social connectedness to peers, and the drug's popularity and availability were mentioned as factors influencing use.[5] It was widely viewed that marijuana was much safer than alcohol or tobacco. Many of the study participants did not consider cannabis to be a drug.[5] When CCSA researchers asked why those surveyed felt this way, their responses included; that it was "natural" (not man-made), "safe" and "non-addictive".[5]

In January of 2017, CCSA released an updated survey: *Canadian Youth Perceptions on Cannabis, outlining current perceptions of Canadian youth on marijuana use: Cannabis isn't harmful.*[6] Most youth in the new study held the view that cannabis is "safe" or does not have significant harms, especially when compared to other substances.[6] (The CCSA in 2017, became the Canadian Centre on Substance Use and Addiction.)

The percentage of children aged 11, 13 and 15 who report having used cannabis in the last 12 months is highest in Canada reported UNICEF in 2013.[7] Only in Norway had the rate of cannabis use by young people fallen below 5%. The young people of six countries recorded cannabis use rates of 20% or more. They were Canada, the Czech Republic, France, Spain, Switzerland and the United States.[7]

"People were not taught the harms of weed until it was too late. But the reality that high THC content is hurting them is through experience and not through the education they should have received."[8] —Harrison Chamberlain, a junior at Golden High School, Colorado (2016)

The decision to participate in illicit drugs is largely driven by a desire to experience the "fashionable" or "celebrated" pastimes of the day, as defined by friends, siblings, or by society at large. In this context, drug use becomes a way of belonging. Deciding to participate in risky activities in order to fit in with school mates, get along with peers, or a significant other, explains why some youth go on to use in spite of having received the "education". It has been well established that peer pressure is especially pronounced and influential during adolescence.

Young children in contrast, prioritize adult views over those of their peers. This does not render adult or parental guidance insignificant for adolescents but does suggest special attention is needed in addressing this demographic in the way prevention messaging is presented.

Parents, with strong views in opposition to drug use, can have a tremendous impact on their child's subsequent rejection of drugs.[9] However, the desire to become involved in a "drug culture" may override parental advice, especially if the information being provided is considered dubious.

IDENTIFYING THE PROBLEM   Youth have been negatively impacted by marijuana propaganda that has consistently downplayed and outright dismissed the warnings of the potential for harm linked to the use of marijuana products.

THEY WANT THEIR POT AND THEY WANT IT NOW *Just Say Now,* lead their website mastheads.[10] Central to the pro-marijuana campaign is the premise that adults deserve the right to private indulgences, specifically the use of marijuana products, without interference by the state. Without due consideration of the costs to the whole of society the marijuana legalization argument rapidly loses credibility. Without an evaluation of the influence and consequences of adult use on the young the argument falls apart.

Smoking or eating marijuana products is not worthy of the status of social activism. For all the flag waving, fanfare and antics of the marijuana revelers, their cause remains stuck in one demand; to get temporarily "high" without legal consequence.

The marijuana debate now constitutes a complicated

discourse over philosophic and political ideology. The highly charged rhetoric, raging across North America over the legalization of drugs, has been heavily influenced by well-funded marijuana activists, some of whom have been working the campaign for decades. By keeping close to a well-honed script "the pot brigade" have been successful in directing the conversation away from the realm of public health. The result of this orchestration is that neither the Canadian populace nor the American people have had the public health conversation they need to have over marijuana policy.

When a law enforcement officer publically announces on a radio talk show that marijuana possession is not a cause for serious concern and that "the war on drugs has failed"; one wonders what a child may be deducing, listening from the back seat of the family car on their way home from school, or from across the room.[10] North American kids have been sold on marijuana, through the media, and by a sophisticated propaganda machine that has been able to reduce the level of concern. This is the insult, which should cost them the ground they seek.

On March 17, 2017, *The Seattle Times* published, *The Case for Eating Weed at Work*, and reported that marijuana producers were getting into the business of making low-dose mints and confectionary products for use during the workday.[11] The marijuana producers claimed that micro-dosing on marijuana products could improve the user's problem-solving abilities, enhance creativity and productivity, and reduce anxiety.[11] Low dose mints and chocolate espresso beans with 5mg THC were reported to be the best sellers.[11] The profiled company's website shows images under the "products" tab for artisan confections such as a "blackberry dark chocolate bars" with 180mg of THC, with a serving size of 45mg of THC.[11] *The Seattle Times'* article did not mention the heightened risk of addiction to marijuana linked to daily use, nor that fat-soluble THC accumulates in body fat stores and tissues, including the brain with unknown consequences.[11]

A major scientific study published by the *Journal of School Health* in July of 2017, reconfirmed what other studies had shown; teenagers who regularly smoke marijuana achieve poorer grades at school and risk their chances of going on to university.[12] The study indicated that for high school students, who started smoking marijuana daily, their likelihood of reporting ambitions to pursue university was around fifty percent lower than for the students who had never used the drug. The longitudinal study of more than 26,400 Canadian students found marijuana users were four times more likely to skip classes and two-to-four times less likely to complete their homework. They also showed less interest in academic achievement.[12]

A study from the University College London suggests that "high" achievers are twice as likely to smoke cannabis during their teenage years due to their curious minds.[13]

The case cannot be made that marijuana is safe, therefore activists campaign on the propaganda that it is "safer" than alcohol, and "safer" than other illicit drugs. The "safer than alcohol" talking point is not a statement of fact but rather a strategic attempt to manipulate the perception of risks. Pot activists also promote the concept of "responsible use".

In June of 2017, an article in *The American Journal of Public Health*; outlined the ways that users could lower their risk of adverse outcomes from marijuana products.[14] Included in the recommendations were calls for abstinence, a delay in initiating use past the age of sixteen and warnings of use in pregnancy. Especially noteworthy was the recommendation that it was "generally preferable" to avoid smoking the drug.[14]

The Canadian Federal Minister for Health issued a media statement applauding the report: "Our Government intends to bring the proposed act (*Bill C-45 The Cannabis Bill*) into force no later than July 2018. It will be important for those who choose to use cannabis for non-medical use to understand how they can minimize the risks of use."[15] Only smoked products would become legal under *Bill C-45*. Edible products would be subject for further review and possible future consideration and legislation.

In 2016, *Vancity Buzz* reported that over sixty people had been admitted to a hospital, requiring treatment for nausea, vomiting, and various states of consciousness, likely from the ingestion of marijuana edible products associated with their having attended the Vancouver 4/20 festivities.[16] In 2017, 4/20 Vancouver-style saw a repeat of the problem, with once again dozens of individuals needing medical attention, with some of the ill as young as 14 years of age.[17] The authorities in Denver, Colorado gave notice to the organizers of Denver 4/20, banning them from holding the event for three years due the property damage caused in 2017.[18] In Vancouver, B.C. the local authorities, in response to extensive damage to a "smoke-free" park, were also faced with considering penalties, fines and the future of 4/20 in the city.

Parks can be repaired, the grass will grow back in. The problem that needs serious attention is how to reverse the enthusiasm many youth and young adults, and a growing number of adults, have for smoking pot.

The Pew Research Center in 2015, found variations in terms of support for legalization; 68% of Millennials thought marijuana should be legal, 29% of the Silent Generation and 50% of Baby Boomers were in favor.[19]

A National Drug Control Policy media conference was held on May 3, 2005 in Washington D.C. under the banner: *Marijuana and Your Teen's Mental Health.*[20] The federal agency sought to alert parents of mental health harms of teens' marijuana use. Mental health experts and scientists joined officials to discuss an emerging body of research that identified clear links between marijuana use and mental health disorders, including depression, suicidal thoughts and schizophrenia. A couple whose 15-year-old committed suicide also presented. The USA Substance Abuse and Mental Health Service Administration (SAMHSA) released a report at the same time that outlined the correlation between age of first marijuana use and serious mental illness.[21]

An open letter to parents and the media, *Marijuana and Your Teen's Mental Health,* signed by twelve of the America's leading mental health organizations, released at the meeting emphasized the risk factors for adolescent marijuana harms: "Regular use of the drug has appeared to double the risk of developing a psychotic episode or long-term schizophrenia. Research has strongly suggested that there is a clear link between early cannabis use and later mental health problems in those with a genetic vulnerability—and that there is a particular issue with the use of cannabis by adolescents. Adolescents who used cannabis daily were five times more likely to develop depression and anxiety in later life."[22] These important announcements were made over 10 years ago.

REWRITING HISTORY Alcohol prohibition (1920–1933) was an attempt to control an already legalized and problematic product. "Analogies with the Prohibition era, often drawn by those who would legalize drugs, are false and inexact: it is one thing to attempt to ban a substance that has been in customary use for centuries by at least nine-tenths of the adult population, and quite another to retain a ban on substances that are still not in customary use, in an attempt to ensure that they never do become customary."[23] Theodore Dalrymple

"Alcohol consumption dropped from 1.96 gallons per person in 1919, to .97 gallons per person in 1934 the first full year after Prohibition ended. Death rates from cirrhosis among men came down from 29.5 per 100,000 in 1911 to 10.7 per 100,000 in 1929. During Prohibition, admission to mental health institutions for alcohol psychosis dropped 60%; arrests for drunk and disorderly conduct went down by 50%; welfare agencies reported significant declines in cases due to alcohol-related family problems; and the death rate from impure alcohol did not rise. Nor did Prohibition generate a crime wave. Homicide increased at a higher rate between 1900 and 1910 than during Prohibition, and organized crime was well established in the cities before 1920."[24] —Joseph A. Califana Jr.

SOMETIMES THE SCIENCE IS FORGOTTEN Sometimes the science is misinterpreted, and sometimes the "tribe" just plain gets the story wrong. A media report in 1991, caused an overnight sensation on the announcement that wine could have health benefits.[25] Dr. Serge Renaud had studied the effects of alcohol on health for 40 years, as the Director of Cardiology at the French National Institute of Health and Medical Research. He appeared on *60 Minutes* (NBC) in 1991 to an audience of 33 million people, to whom he reported that alcohol, specifically red wine, could reduce the risks of heart disease. In the month following the program, sales of red wine increased by 2.5 million bottles in the USA. The episode was replayed in 1992, and the sale of red wine went up by 49% for the month. The doctor also called for a total prohibition on binge drinking and suggested that the amount of alcohol that was potentially beneficial needed was merely a sniff.[25] The public heard what they wanted to hear.

The IARC's *World Cancer Report* of 2014 and the Canadian Cancer Society both state that there is no "safe limit" of alcohol consumption when it comes to cancer prevention.[26]

THE UNDER-REPORTED   In June of 2017, UNICEF released *Poor health, violence at alarming rates among Canada's kids.*[27] Canada had been found to be lagging farthest behind other countries concerning indicators of child health and violence, including child homicide cases.[27] The report showed that Canadian teen mental health has been declining, with 22% of adolescents in Canada reporting mental health symptoms more than once a week and that Canada ranks 31st out of 41 countries in the teen suicide rate.[27]

The UNICEF report is a call for serious review of what a generation of young people and their parents are learning about marijuana harms. It is also a call for far greater efforts to be made, including by all levels of government, to address marijuana use and mental illnesses.

Going from an occasional user of marijuana to a weekly

or daily user increases an adolescent's risk of having recurrent psychotic-like experiences by 159%, according to a Canadian study published July 5, 2017, in *The Journal of Child Psychology and Psychiatry.*[28] Psychotic-like experiences are defined as, experiences of perceptual aberration, ideas with unusual content and feelings of persecution.[28] The study's lead author, Josiane Bourque, a doctoral student at Université de Montréal's Department of Psychiatry reports: "Our findings confirm that becoming a more regular marijuana user during adolescence is, indeed, associated with a risk of psychotic symptoms. This is a major public-health concern for Canada."[29]

"Vulnerability to harmful effects of marijuana appears to be even more pronounced for youth poised to interact with psychiatric and other mental health care treatment providers because of the existence of neuropsychiatric risk factors. This combination of facts suggests that there is a momentous 'storm' coming towards us of upcoming need for psychiatric and addictions services that we have no clear way to adequately meet or prevent. As providers of care, this should be of concern."[30] —Elizabeth Osuch, M.D., FRCPC, ABPN

"Neither nature, human evolution, nor fate created the new burdens of chronic diseases and injuries. Rather, it was human decisions made in corporate boardrooms, advertising and lobbying firms, and legislative and judicial chambers."[31] —Nicholas Freudenberg, D.P. Public Health

1. A Wake Up Call

"We believed that an informed electorate would be generally opposed if they knew the facts. The overall message after being informed about this marijuana, was that it is not safe, and that it is harmful."[1] —James Otten. In November of 2014, a referendum was put to a Denver, Colorado suburb, which if successful would block the growing, distribution and retailing of marijuana within the city limits of Lakewood. James Otten, who was instrumental in the campaign discussed the results: "In 2012, Lakewood voters favored legalizing recreational pot by a 55-45 margin. But last year, they voted 54-46 to block it in their community."[2]

"It's not worth it," Colorado Attorney General Cynthia Coffman told assembled state attorney generals, at a conference in Washington D.C. in February of 2015, in reference to the millions being collected in taxes from pot sales in the State of Colorado.[3] "The criminals are still selling on the black market. We have plenty of cartel activity in Colorado and plenty of illegal action that has not decreased at all," said Coffman.[3]

Dr. David F. Musto (1936-2010), credited the observation of the damage caused by drugs as the primary catalyst for triggering declines in use.[4,5] Surveys on the perception of risk from the mid-1980s show a connection was in fact made with a risk of marijuana harms after more than a decade of high levels of use.[6]

In 1978, 10.7% of high school students in the United States were smoking marijuana products every day.[6] The use of marijuana peaked in 1979, followed by a period of dramatic decline between 1979 and 1992 for past month use, past year use and lifetime use.[6] By 1985, 7 out of 10 high school seniors considered marijuana products to be harmful.[6] In1992, the rate of high school students who smoked marijuana products daily dropped below 2%.[6]

By 1980, a co-ordinated parent movement had emerged in reaction to the high prevalence of use, as well as to the explosive rise of a "drug culture" and to the observed damage of which Dr. Musto wrote. Throughout the late 1970s and the 1980s, concerned parents would became a recognized force with significant political power. The Parent Movement supported decision makers who were willing to take action on the drug crisis and they would get the results they were pushing for during the presidency of Ronald Reagan. "Between 1979 and 1991, a huge prevention campaign in America coincided with a dramatic decrease in drug use. Parents, teachers, police, youth leaders, social workers, churches, the children themselves, all got involved—it worked. Users fell from 23 to 14 million. Cannabis and cocaine use halved, daily cannabis use dropped 75%."[7] —Mary Brett (UK).

Those who claim prohibition as a public health strategy is not effectual either do not know or have forgotten the narcotics record for the period of the 1970s through to 1992 in the United States. For all the valuable information from the world of science, the evidence from the historical record can also be relied on to lead the direction of drug policy. Canada and the United States have succeeded in reducing rates of marijuana use in the past and results were achieved once a course that relied on prevention rather than on harm minimization strategies was set.

Today, individuals continue to work on behalf of families through organization such as Parents Opposed to Pot, Moms Strong, and Smart Approaches to Marijuana in the United States and in Canada, Citizens against Legalizing Marijuana (CALM-California), along with many others in North America and around the world. A list of non-profit organizations working to build communities that are free of marijuana and/or other illegal drugs is at *The Marijuana Report*: http:themarijuanareport.org

The changes to federal drug policy, brought in during the Reagan administration, were strongly opposed by marijuana activists. Rather than lessen restrictions, American society moved to a tightening of drug policies. The Reagan era would come to be known for the *Just Say No* campaign and for a tough on drugs stance.

Reefer Madness was a doctored version of a 1936 film titled, *Tell Your Children*. The parent-church group who funding the original production did so in an attempt to dissuade young people from using drugs. It was re-edited to become a trashy exploitation film that took on the off-limits subject of drug use and it went on to play on the underground theatre film circuit in order to circumvent the 1930 *Motion Picture Production Code*. The code had made it illegal to depict drug trafficking and activity in any way that would stimulate curiosity, or show scenes of the use of illicit drugs.

The government of the USA had no involvement with either *Tell Your Children* or *Reefer Madness*, nor did the FBI or any other federal agency. *Reefer Madness* was revived in the early 1970s by Keith Stroup of NORML (National Organization for the Reform of Marijuana Laws) and toured around university campuses to finance the newly-formed pro-marijuana organization. The term *Reefer Madness* is deployed today by marijuana activists, used as a ready attack against those that stand in their way and by those who view warnings of marijuana harms as mere government generated propaganda, as hysteria or a threat to their self-proclaimed "movement".

THE CANADIAN GAMBLE Marijuana policy was included in policy discussions during the 2015 national election in Canada. Prime Minister Justin Trudeau made the legalization of marijuana for non-medical use part of his campaign rhetoric. Legalization was also a ratified policy the Liberal Party of Canada. The Trudeau majority government reiterated in 2017 that they considered such a significant change in public health policy within their mandate, in spite of the issue not having been a priority issue for the general electorate before, during or after the election.

A federally appointed Canadian task force, charged with drafting a regulatory framework for the legalization of marijuana issued a public discussion paper in June of 2016 and invited input from Canadians. They received some 30,000 responses in a country of 36.5 million people.[8]

Today, millions of school-age Canadian children are using marijuana on a regular basis. With such a large number of school-age children using marijuana products, Canadian families must be experiencing the problems that follow marijuana use, especially by those addicted or using on a regular basis.

Data from 2009-2010 shows that approximately 28% of Canadians aged 15 and older who used cannabis in the past three months had used this drug every day or almost every day.[9] The number of youth, who had used cannabis within the year, was three times higher than the number of Canadians aged 25 years and older (21.6% vs. 6.7%) and in some jurisdictions, approximately 50% of grade 12 students reported consuming cannabis within the year.[9] In excess of 6% of Canadian high school seniors reported smoking marijuana on a daily basis in 2014.[10] As the addiction rate for marijuana users is 1 in 2 for daily users, 1 in 6 for regular youth users, the Canadian youth use rates are alarming. [11,12]

THE AMERICAN GAMBLE A 2012–2013 Colorado report documents why 720 students were expelled from public schools across the state.[13] Marijuana was the reason for 32% of all student expulsions.[13] The Colorado Education Association, the state's largest union of teachers, opposed *Amendment 64, Regulate Marijuana like Alcohol*, as did the CEA Board of Directors.[14]

"Regular marijuana use by adolescents is associated with low academic achievement, such as not graduating from high school."[15] —Oregon Health Authority 2016 "When one in five high school youth is regularly using a substance known to impair cognitive performance, at stronger and stronger dose levels and increasingly with a pattern a daily consumption, the impact could well be sufficient to change society."[16] —The Hudson Institute, USA

REVISITING A DECISION   The USA Drug Enforcement Administration (DEA) in 1989 released a ruling that denied a petition from the National Organization for the Reform of Marijuana Law (NORML). NORML had pursued a reclassification of marijuana from a Schedule I to a Schedule II. A Schedule I drug, substance or chemical is given this classification if it has no current accepted medical use and has a high potential for abuse. Schedule II drugs, substances or chemicals are given this classification if they have a high potential for abuse, with their use potentially leading to severe psychological or physical dependence.

Opposed to the rescheduling included the DEA, the National Federation of Parents for a Drug-Free Youth, and the International Association of Chiefs of Police. Several key passages from the 1989 ruling, as published by the *Federal Register, Vol. 54, No 249*, read as follows: "The evidence presented by the pro-marijuana parties include outdated and limited scientific studies; chronicles of individuals, their families and friends who have used marijuana; opinions from over a dozen psychiatrists and physicians; court opinions involving medical necessity as a defense to criminal charges for illegal possession of marijuana; state statues which made marijuana available for research; newspaper articles; and the opinions of laypersons, including lawyers and associations of lawyers.

The Administrator does not find such evidence convincing in light of the lack of reliable, credible, and relevant scientific studies documenting marijuana's utility; the opinions of highly respected, credentialed experts that marijuana does not have an accepted medical use; and statements from the American Medical Association, the American Cancer Society, the American Academy of Ophthalmology, the National Multiple Sclerosis Society, and the Federal Food and Drug Administration that marijuana has not been demonstrated as suitable for use as a medicine. The ruling listed one hundred finding of facts that supported the decision.

As a final note, the Administrator expresses his displeasure at the misleading accusations and conclusions leveled at the Government and communicated to the public by the pro-marijuana parties, specifically NORML and ACT (Alliance for Cannabis Therapeutics). These two organizations have falsely raised the expectations of many seriously ill persons by claiming that marijuana has medical usefulness in treating emesis, glaucoma, spasticity and other illnesses. These statements have probably caused many people with serious diseases to experiment with marijuana to the detriment to their own health, without proper medical supervision, and without knowledge about the serious side effects which smoking or ingesting marijuana may cause. These are not the Dark Ages.

The Congress, as well as the medical community, has accepted that drugs should not be available to the public unless they are found by scientific studies to be effective and safe. To do otherwise is to jeopardize the American public, and take advantage of the desperately ill people who will try anything to alleviate their suffering. The Administrator strongly urges the American public not to experiment with a potentially dangerous, mind-altering drug such as marijuana in an attempt to treat serious illness or condition.

Scientific and medical researchers are working tirelessly to develop treatments and drugs to treat these diseases and conditions....NORML and ACT have attempted to perpetrate a dangerous and cruel hoax on the American public by claiming marijuana has currently accepted medical uses. The Administration again emphasizes that there is insufficient medical and scientific evidence to support a conclusion that marijuana has an accepted medical use for treatment for any condition, or that it is safe for use, even under medical supervision."[17] This important letter could have been written in 2017. The contents remain not only valid but also relevant.

Science released through the 1970s significantly advanced the understanding of both short and long term effects associated with marijuana. In 1970, researchers at the US National Institute of Mental Health determined that marijuana metabolites remain in the body for days after use; accumulating in certain tissues and organs for extended periods of time.[18] The finding that fat-soluble marijuana impacts the human body differently than water soluble alcohol sparked a new interest in scientific study on marijuana in relation to health.[19]

In 1975, at an international gathering of pharmacologists in Helsinki, Finland, the attendees learned of current research conducted by Cecile Leuchtenberger. This research demonstrated that when cells from testis were exposed to marijuana smoke they had a marked decrease in DNA, compared to those exposed to tobacco smoke.[20] These results suggested serious reproductive consequences if, in fact, marijuana smoke resulted in the formation of abnormal cells.[20] Now, more than 40 years since the Leuchtenberger research, with advances in the science of reproductive health, public health agencies caution women if pregnant, and men planning on starting a family to avoid the use of marijuana products.[21]

Current scientific research suggests that women also avoid

marijuana products pre-conception.[22] "Women who smoke marijuana either prior to or during pregnancy may also do other risky behaviours, like maybe drink alcohol and maybe partake in other illicit drugs. What our data analysis has shown, though, is that marijuana has independent effects."[23] —Professor Clair Roberts. Research shows marijuana use is particularly harmful for women in the three months before pregnancy.[23] The DEA ruling of 1989 was the correct decision.

A 1985 study, published in the *American Journal of Psychiatry*, found ten pilots, each given one "social-dose" marijuana cigarette (with 20mg of THC), had trouble flying a simulation machine.[24] Seven of the pilots showed impaired performance a day after the test, with only one pilot cognizant that he remained impaired.[24] "These results suggest concern for performance of those entrusted with complex behavioral and cognitive tasks within 24 hours after smoking marijuana," said Dr. Jerome Yesavage.[25] Scientific studies show that cognitive and psychomotor functions are impaired directly after cannabis use and impairment can persist for several days.[26]

Canada in 2012: Marijuana collisions amounted to 75 deaths and 4407 injuries; 24,789 people were victims of property damage from "marijuana-only" collisions.[27] The marijuana collision costs ranged from $1.09 to $1.28 billion CDN for the year.[27] The report was made public in 2017, but was vastly under-reported.

WARNING There is substantial evidence that for a less-than-weekly user to eat one small gummy candy product, with 10mg of THC, it is likely their driving ability will be meaningfully impaired. There is substantial evidence that following consumption of 1.8 parts of a gummy candy (18mg), a less-than-weekly user should not drive for a minimum of 8 hours.[28] (Marijuana infused gummy candies made in the shape of bears, or other animals, fruits or people were made illegal in Colorado in October of 2016, as regulators determined they were far too attractive to children.[29])

Lives have been lost due to the use of marijuana products, and this fact seldom if ever makes the headlines at the time of the accidents, as toxicology reports and investigations are lengthy processes. This disconnect is only part of the problem. The public has been bombarded with messaging that purports that the worst possible outcome that can be inflicted on the individual user, if caught in possession by law enforcement, is that they could see their international travel curtailed or job prospects reduced.[30] This is a serious under-statement of the potential of harms, including accidents, in the home, on the job site and on roadways.

In 2016, Mario Cortez was sentenced to 40 years in prison after he killed a couple while driving with five times the Nevada legal limit of marijuana in his blood. The victims were both in their mid-70s.[31]

In 2014, prosecutors decided that NASCAR driving champion Tony Stewart would not be charged with the death of a fellow driver. The prosecutors disclosed that the victim had enough marijuana in his system at the time of the accident to impair his judgement. The individual was killed when he got out of his own vehicle and was hit by the car Stewart was driving.[32]

Haven Dubois, a 14-year-old boy died in May of 2015. His body was pulled from a creek near his home in east Regina, Saskatchewan, Canada. The coroner's report stated the cause of death was drowning with marijuana as a contributing factor.[33] Included in the coroner's report were interviews with the boy's friends, who related that they skipped a school job fair the day he died and started smoking marijuana. They described Haven's reaction to marijuana as "freaking out."[33] A friend reported that he had walked with Haven to a park and left him sitting on a bench while he went back to the high school to get his friend's backpack and skateboard. When he returned, Haven was gone. The report says another friend went to Haven's home and told someone there that he had seen him walking by the creek. That's when his mother began to search. No one to date has been charged for providing the drugs that contributed to Haven's death.

There are those who would have the public believe the marijuana deaths having nothing to do with marijuana use but rather the fall was "gravity", the crash a case of "bad driving", the downed plane —"the weather" and Haven's death—well that was just a case of drowning. What they fail to accept is Haven knew how to swim, the pilot was stoned, and the fall was induced by a psychiatric reaction to high potency marijuana. Coroner's toxicology reports tell the real story, as do family members and witnesses at horrific events.

The argument that impaired driving is merely "bad driving" is no longer a defense. Marijuana has now been implicated and attributed to the deaths of many a victim and the argument that marijuana has never resulted in dire consequences, including death, is insulting to the memory of those that have lost their lives after being sold on marijuana, as it is to those innocent bystanders who were killed by the actions of an impaired person, as it is to their grieving, shattered families.

2. A Trojan Horse

Remedy Ice Cream is produced and distributed out of Alberta, Canada. It consists of ice-cream that has been infused with high potency THC —"shatter".[1] The producers claim the product is for licensed medical marijuana patients only and that they ask for a driver's license and a medical prescription. The company does not have a license to sell this product, however they publically discuss their enterprise and they have an online presence through which they promote their product and handle sales. The product is shipped in dry ice across the country.[1]

"This is the greatest hoax of all time," commented Michael Bloomberg, the former Mayor of New York City answering a request for his comment on marijuana legalization by *CBC News* in 2013.[2]

In 1979, Keith Stroup of NORML gave a presentation to Emory University: "We will use the medical marijuana argument as a red herring on the road to full legalization."[3] His successor Richie Cowan, at a 1993 conference: "Medical marijuana is our strongest suit. It is our point of leverage which will move us towards the legalization of marijuana for personal use."[4] After the *Compassionate Use Act* passed in California in 1996, Allen St. Pierre, the director of NORML, admitted in a CNN TV interview that: "In California marijuana has also been de facto legalized under the guise of medical marijuana."[5]

In June 2015, an editorial in *The Journal of the American Medical Association* (*JAMA*) argued there was little evidence to support marijuana for medical use: "First, for most qualifying conditions, approval has relied on low-quality scientific evidence, anecdotal reports, individual testimonies, legislative initiatives, and public opinion."[6] The *JAMA* editorial also mentioned that patients were suffering from side effects, from the use of cannabis, with disturbing frequency.[6]

On June 28, 2015, *The Denver Post* responded to the *JAMA* editorial with an editorial titled; *The Moment of truth for medical Marijuana:* "With so little scientific evidence that medical marijuana does what it purported to do, it may be time to retire the medical model—at least in states like Colorado where marijuana can be legally purchased by an adult."[7] The editors also noted that there remains no solid scientific evidence of benefit for the list of "debilitating medical conditions" that had been included in *Amendment 20* that had legalized medi-pot marijuana for residents of Colorado in 2000.[7]

The Oregon Public Health Authority in 2011, saw a small proportion of medical marijuana users reporting use for cancer or HIV/AIDS or glaucoma; 4% for cancer, 2% for HIV/AIDS and 1% for glaucoma.[8] In Colorado, 2% reported using for cancer, less than 1% reporting for HIV/AIDS or glaucoma.[9]

In April of 2015, the Governor of Idaho wrote to the Secretary of State for Idaho: "I hereby advise you that I have returned without my approval and vetoed the following *Senate Bill, to wit: S1146a.* I do not know what more I or senior members of my administration could have done to help legislators understand our strong opposition to this legislation. Both the House and the Senate were told by the Office of Drug Policy, the Department of Health and Welfare, and the Idaho State Police—as well as prosecutors and local law enforcement officers from throughout Idaho—that there were too many questions and problems and too few answers and solutions in this bill to become law.

Of course I sympathize with the heartbreaking dilemma facing some families trying to cope with the debilitating impacts of disease. They find themselves grasping for an answer—any answer that might help reduce or eliminate the pain and suffering, or that might provide some hope for a better, healthier future. It is difficult as a public official to separate those very real and profoundly upsetting situations from the tough public policy decisions we are elected to make. Nonetheless, such separation sometimes is necessary.

From the purposefully incorrect fiscal impact statement to the claims of patient outcomes that are more speculative than scientific, this legislation unfortunately—and with the very best of intentions and sense of humanity—is not what Benjamin Franklin meant when he described states as the laboratories of the republic. It ignores ongoing scientific testing on alternative treatments. It asks us to trust but not to verify. It asks us to legalize the limited use of cannabidiol oil, contrary to federal law and it asks us to look past the potential for misuse and abuse with criminal intent.

So in vetoing this legislation, I echo the sentiments of the administers of my Office of Drug Policy and the director of Health and Welfare, who wrote in an April 7 letter to me: 'While we acknowledge the compassionate intention of *S1146a*, the list of negative outcomes associated with this bill will be extensive in our quest to relieve suffering, it is vital that we insure the solutions employed do not exacerbate health problems for the critically ill or decrease public safety. This bill has the potential to do both.'

As an alternative to this legislation, I soon will issue an Executive Order authorizing the Department of Health and Welfare to study, and implement as it deems appropriate, an expanded access program for treatment –resistant epilepsy in children. That program has been approved by the U.S. Food and Drug Administration." —"As Always—Idaho, "Esto Perpetua" C.L. "Butch" Otter Governor of Idaho."[10]

Idaho's Governor, Butch Otter is the only United States governor to have vetoed a medi-pot bill. Governor Otter created an expanded Epidiolex program that has benefitted numerous children and advanced the cause of medical research. Patients have been given experimental drugs under *The Compassionate Care Act*, and their progress is being studied. Providing scientifically unproven drugs to any patient, while exposing the vast population to mixed and potentially dangerous messaging about these substances, is a serious issue that must be reconciled.

"The world is watching Washington's historic experiment with marijuana legalization, and we're screwing it up.... Medical marijuana dispensaries appear to outnumber Starbuck stores in Seattle, yet local regulators and law-enforcement agencies are doing almost nothing to police bad actors hiding behind the ubiquitous green crosses."[11] —*The Seattle Times*, 2014

"Stings caught three of 10 licensed marijuana stores in Pierce County, and two of eight in Thurston County selling to minors, state regulators say. The agency soon to be renamed the Liquor and Cannabis Board made its first round of checks for sales to minors in May and June, sending 18- to 20-year-olds into shops to buy pot."[12] —Jordan Schrader, *the News Tribune* (2015)

"At the end of the day, all the arguments for legalization of marijuana have yet to be convincing. The best argument is the one which goes unspoken: some individuals simply want the right to get stoned, free of potential legal consequences, and without concern as to whether that right would carry a likelihood of harm for either themselves or others. Where we not living in a society where we each have responsibility for one another's health and welfare, perhaps such an argument would rule the day."[13] —Dr. Stuart Gitlow.

On November 25, 2014 Health Canada issued warning letters to 20 licensed producers regarding their advertising practices.[14] The warning letters followed up an advertising bulletin that had been sent to all licensed producers in June that outlined the general prohibitions against the advertising of marijuana contained in the *Marijuana for Medical Purposes Regulations*, the *Food and Drugs Act* and the *Narcotic Control Regulations*. The warning read: "The licensees are to limit the information they share with the public to basis information such as brand name, proper and common name of the strain, price per gram, the cannabinoid content, and the company's contact details."[14]

The government was concerned about marijuana producers' marketing practises and serious errors and omissions about the therapeutic use of cannabis, of its contradictions and dosing. Claims were being made that dried cannabis may be beneficial for a variety of conditions. Some of the producer's websites referred to research that had been done on marijuana but they failed to state that this research was preliminary, uncontrolled, or pre-clinical and some of the claims made by licensees contravened the *Canadian Food and Safety Act*, which prohibits claims of therapeutic benefit for specific medical conditions. Many of the licensee websites also failed to provide a comprehensive list of contraindications and precautions prior to use.[15]

Doctors practising in the United States cannot "*prescribe*" marijuana in any state, as no marijuana product that has been "legalized" by a state government is legal under federal law. To circumvent federal law, states authorize doctors to "recommend" marijuana to patients or to certify that a patient has a qualifying condition. The December 2016 (The American Bar Association), *Health Lawyer Newsletter,* published a report outlining potential consequences doctors could face if federal law is enforced.[16]

Two of the chemicals in marijuana are Tetrahydrocannabinol (THC) and Cannabidiol (CBD). THC is responsible for the psychoactive effect and CBD has antipsychotic, and anti-anxiety properties. The ratio of THC to CBD is being manipulated by today's producers to provide their customers with a greater "high". These higher potency products are known to increase the risk of addiction.

THC is fat-soluble and goes directly to the brain. A minimal amount resides in the blood stream following smoking or eating edible products. The plant contains at least 750 chemicals, with some 104 different cannabinoids. CBD is now being produced as an "artisan" grade product and is also being researched as a pharmaceutical grade drug.

THE MISUSE OF SCIENCE TO PUSH MARIJUANA   Over thirty years ago the pharmaceutical industry took a serious interest in the marijuana plant. Researchers picked up on anecdotal evidence on the efficacy of marijuana in relation to alleviating nausea. Their hope was that part of the marijuana plant might be used for the development of new medications, specifically for the relief of chemotherapy induced vomiting and nausea. Researchers were able to isolate THC, and establish this chemical's efficacy for the relief of chemotherapy induced vomiting and nausea.[17] They were also able to identify a corresponding side effect profile.[17]

The science of pharmacological drug production depends on the capability of scientists to isolate individual chemicals and replicate them in synthetic form. Through this process, they can eliminate potentially toxic, possibly deadly molds, fungi, carcinogens, formaldehyde, contaminates, and other chemicals in the primary substance that could cause adverse effects or negatively interact with other medications. The more isolated the chemical, the purer the product. The more consistent the substance is in terms of dosage, and what is known of its pharmacokinetics (absorption, distribution, and elimination), its side effect profile and how it interacts with other drugs, foods, etc., the safer the product.

In 1985, the orally active dronabinol (Marinol), a synthetic THC pharmaceutical grade derived product, was granted FDA approval.[18] The approval was for the specific use in chemotherapy induced vomiting and nausea in for patients who failed to respond adequately to conventional antiemetic regimens, namely anorexia associated with weight loss and for patients with AIDS. Nabilone (Cessamet) is another synthetic cannabinoid approved by the FDA in 1985, solely for the use in nausea and vomiting associated with chemotherapy. Both drugs are now so old that they are available as generic products (no longer solely sold under the original trade name and have lost U.S. patent exclusivity).

By the 1990s and 2000s, the pharmaceutical industry had moved on to better drugs with less side effects for the condition of chemotherapy induced nausea and vomiting with the 5-HT3 (serotonin) receptor antagonists (i.e. ondansetron (Zofran), granisetron (Kytril, etc.) and neurokinin 1 receptor antagonists (i.e. aprepitant (Emend oral), fosaprepitant (Emend injection). Dronabinol has fallen out of favor for chemotherapy induced nausea and vomiting primarily due to its adverse effect profile with limited efficacy. In the most recent *American Society of Clinical Oncology's (ASCO) Antiemetic Guidelines* dronabinol is listed as an adjunct to those who have failed serotonin antagonists or steroids and neurokinin antagonists.[19]

Since 1985, no other marijuana derived pharmaceutical products was developed by the multi-billion dollar pharmaceutical industry until the recent GW Pharmaceutical's scientific investigations into cannabidiol (CBD). CBD may have a role in treating rare and serious forms of epilepsy in children— Dravet Syndrome and Lennox-Gastaut Syndrome.[20]

On March 14 of 2016, GW Pharmaceuticals announced a positive result for their Phase 3 Study of CBD in the treatment of Dravet Syndrome.[21] Representatives of the company stated that their medicine had achieved a high statistical significance showing their drug treatment reduced convulsive seizures in children enrolled in the study, compared to placebo.[21] Their brand drug product had previously received both *Orphan*

Drug Designation and *Fast Track Designation* from the FDA and there is currently no FDA treatment for the disorder. The pharmaceutical product currently in clinical trials is a synthetic derivative from the marijuana plant. It may prove to be of great benefit to the children suffering with this serious and life threatening condition.

The Phase 3 Study randomized 120 patients into two arms, Epidiolex (CBD) 20 mg/kg/day (n = 61) and placebo (n = 59). Epidiolex or placebo was added to current anti-epileptic drug treatment programs. The average age of trial participants was 10 years old and 30% of patients were less than 6 years of age. The median baseline convulsive seizure frequency of the participants per month was 13.[21]

The primary efficacy endpoint was a comparison between Epidiolex and placebo measuring the percentage change in the monthly frequency of convulsive seizures during the 14-week treatment period compared with the 4-week baseline observation period. In this study, patients taking Epidiolex achieved a median reduction in monthly convulsive seizures of 39% compared with a reduction on placebo of 13%.[21]

The most common adverse events were somnolence, diarrhea, decreased appetite, fatigue, pyrexia, vomiting, lethargy, upper respiratory tract infections and convulsions. Of those participants on Epidiolex that reported an adverse event, 84 % said it was mild or moderate. Ten patients on Epidiolex experienced a serious adverse event compared with three patients on placebo. Eight of the participants on Epidiolex discontinued treatment due to adverse events compared, one patient on placebo discontinued the treatment.[21]

For the most part the pharmaceutical industry has given a pass to the marijuana plant. There are other drugs (including those that have placed HIV infections into the realm of a chronic disease) that surpass the efficacy or need of the one derived from marijuana to date.

With hundreds of chemicals inherent in marijuana, it is not feasible to determine the use of the whole plant as a "safe" medicine. In the interest of patient safety the whole plant is not a recommended medicine by any medical authority; the interaction of its various components are not understood and it is impossible to dose a product with hundreds of various chemicals. Future prospects, in terms of new pharmaceutical grade marijuana products, must come from derivatives of the plant and not the whole plant itself. This is the same for poppies, periwinkle, and all other botanicals that have provided the world with drugs that have saved lives, not from chewing or smoking the whole plant but rather from specific chemicals (opium and vinca alkaloids) within the plants. It is not for a lack of funding or will of trying.

Marijuana interests used the science that launched dronabinol, embellished the claims of benefit of CBD and THC, downplayed or denied the adverse effects. They launched a campaign to get "patients" their "medicine", without the evidence of science, in an age of modern medicine and they played on compassion.

"Smoked marijuana creates 3,000 molecular entities that defy categorization and quantification. If you can't have a known starting point for a drug, measuring its outcome is futile."[22] —Ed Wood, DUID Victim's Voices.

3. The Science

The Health Effects of Cannabis and Cannabinoids 2017 —The Current State of Evidence and Recommendations for Research Committee on the Health Effects of Marijuana, issued by the National Academies of Sciences, Engineering and Medicine (USA), provides a survey of scientific evidence on marijuana use and related conditions and outcomes:

There is substantial evidence of a statistical association between cannabis smoking and worse respiratory symptoms and more frequent chronic bronchitis episodes (long-term cannabis smoking); substantial evidence of a statistical association between cannabis use and an increased risk of motor vehicle crashes; substantial evidence of a statistical association between cannabis use and the development of schizophrenia or other psychoses, with the highest risk among the most frequent users; substantial evidence of a statistical association between maternal cannabis smoking and lower birth weight of the offspring. There is substantial evidence that initiating cannabis use at an earlier age is a risk factor for the development of problem cannabis use; substantial evidence of a statistical association between increases in cannabis use frequency and the progression to developing problem cannabis use; moderate evidence of a statistical association between cannabis use and increased risk of overdose injuries, including respiratory distress, among pediatric populations in U.S. states where cannabis is legal; moderate evidence of a statistical association between cannabis use and increased symptoms of mania and hypomania in individuals diagnosed with bipolar disorders (regular cannabis use). There is limited evidence of cannabis use and increased severity of posttraumatic stress disorder symptoms, moderate evidence of increased risk of the development of substance dependence and/or a substance abuse disorder for substances including, alcohol, tobacco, and other illicit drugs; moderate evidence that during adolescence the frequency of cannabis use, oppositional behaviors, a younger age of first alcohol use, nicotine use, parental substance use, poor school performance, antisocial behaviors, and childhood sexual abuse are risk factors for the development of problem cannabis use.[1]

THE ARGUMENT OVER GATEWAY The June 2016 discussion paper released by the Canadian legalization task force reads: "Marijuana has often been dubbed the 'gateway drug'— a stop on the way to the use of more harmful drugs and more serious drug addiction. The so-called 'gateway hypothesis' was popular in the 1970s/80s and neatly described a specific, progressive and hierarchical sequence of stages of drug use that begins with the use of a 'softer drug' (e.g., marijuana) and escalates to use of 'harder drugs' (e.g., cocaine). However, over the years, many exceptions to and problems with the 'gateway hypothesis' have surfaced. Because of this, the validity and relevance of this hypothesis have been challenged. There is now evidence that suggests that complex interactions among various individual/ predisposing factors and environmental factors (e.g., peer-pressure, family influence, drug availability, opportunities for drug use) drive drug seeking, drug use/abuse, and drug addiction, and these interactions are not necessarily tied to marijuana use alone."[2]

A research paper, presented at the Cannabis and Health International Drug Policy Symposium in Auckland, New Zealand in 2013, chiefly authored by Dr. Wayne Hall, outlined the research results from 1993-2013 in regards to the adverse health effects of recreational marijuana use.[3] The science showed that regular cannabis use in adolescence is associated strongly with the use of other illicit drugs.[3, 4]

The World Health Organization (WHO), through its Department of Mental Health and Substance Abuse, held a meeting in April of 2015 to review and summarize the available knowledge on the effects of nonmedical cannabis use—on health and psychosocial functioning. A WHO document from the meeting reads: "Growing evidence reveals that regular, heavy cannabis use during adolescence is associated with more severe and persistent negative outcomes than use during adulthood. Negative outcomes include: early school-leaving, cognitive impairment, increased risk of using other illicit drugs, increased risk of depressive symptoms, increased rates of suicidal ideation and behaviour. It remains to be determined which of these associations are causal."[5]

Researchers studying at the University of Bristol in June of 2017 reported that regular and occasional marijuana use by teens was associated with a greater risk of other drug use by early adulthood.[6] They also concluded that one in five marijuana using adolescents was at risk for problematic drinking and the use of tobacco products.[6]

"Research shows that the earlier a teen first uses drugs, the likelier he or she is to become addicted to them or to become addicted to another substance later in life."[7] —*Brain In Progress: Why Teens Can't Always Resist Temptation*, Nora Volkow, Director of the National Institute on Drug Abuse, USA, 2015.

THE SCIENCE TOO FEW TALK ABOUT The editors of *Psychology Magazine* in March of 2016, published an article by R. Douglas Fields, Ph.D., entitled *Marijuana Use Increases Violent Behavior, 50 year study finds causal link between cannabis and subsequent violent behavior.*[8] The study discussed in the article was *Continuity of cannabis use and violent offending over the life course*; a study of 411 young males designed to investigate the association between marijuana use and violent behavior.[8] The results showed that continued cannabis use was associated with 7-fold greater odds for subsequent commission of violent crimes and that impairments in neurological circuits controlling behavior may underlie impulsive, violent behavior, as a result of cannabis altering the normal neural functioning in the ventrolateral prefrontal cortex. The results showed a strong indication that marijuana use predicts subsequent violent offending, suggesting a possible causal effect.[8]

The link to marijuana use and increased violence is a vastly neglected discussion in the public debate over whether or not the commercialization of marijuana products is in the best interest of all of society.

Kristine Kirk was shot and killed by her husband. Kristine Kirk had called 911 to report that her husband was hallucinating as a result of taking marijuana candies that he had purchased at a marijuana dispensary. Lawsuits filed in Colorado courts associated with the death claimed that the marijuana businesses involved in the sale of the marijuana used by Mr. Kirk should be found responsible by the courts for her death.[9] The plaintiffs claimed the marijuana product should have carried a warning of the possible side effects, specifically a warning of hallucination, risk of paranoia or marijuana induced psychosis. It was suggested that a warning of the marijuana products potential adverse interaction with other substances should also have been provided at the time of purchase.[9]

As a result of this widely publicized event, warning statements on the side effects were mandated and enforced on edible marijuana products in the state of Colorado in the fall of 2016. The Colorado Department of Revenue requires that all marijuana product packaging display the letters THC in red along with an exclamation mark also in red. The symbol must be stamped onto edible products where possible.

For information on regulations in Colorado the government website is: goodtoknowcolorado.com

The Journal of The American Medicine Association (JAMA) on August 31, 2016 published; *Parental Psychiatric Disease and Risks of Attempted Suicide and Violent Criminal Offending in Offspring. A Population-based Cohort Study.* The study had found that elevated risks of both attempted suicide and violent offending in offspring were evident across a broad spectrum of parental psychiatric disease, with the links being strongest in relation to parental antisocial personality disorder, cannabis misuse, and attempted suicide.[10] The study emphasized that interventions that aim to reduce the incidence of parental substance misuse may help to reduce their offspring's future risks of suicidality and violence. The researchers examined 1,743,525 cohort members with a total follow up of 27.2 million person years (30 years).[10]

In 2013, the international media reported on the findings of the 1993-2013 scientific literature review led by Dr. Wayne Hall. The findings that cannabis-impaired driving approximately doubles car crash risk and regular cannabis use in adolescence doubles the risk of early school leaving were widely reported.[3] In the section of the report on the association with cannabis and cancer, a study is cited that found a doubling of the risk of lung cancer among study subjects who had smoked cannabis fifty or more times by the age of 18. The conclusion was drawn that more study would need to be done to better understand the risks of lung cancer in the cannabis smoking population.[3,11]

"Our primary finding provides initial longitudinal evidence that cannabis use might elevate the risk of lung cancer."[12] —*Cancer Causes & Control,* 2013

In *Marijuana Smoke Contains Higher Levels of Certain Toxins than Tobacco Smoke (2007),* the American Chemical Society reported that scientists found ammonia levels 20 times higher in marijuana smoke than in the tobacco smoke, while hydrogen cyanide, nitric oxide and certain aromatic amines occurring at levels 3–5 times higher in marijuana smoke.[13]

Scientific literature reviews, such as the one conducted by Dr. Wayne Hall, establishes that there is a significant body of epidemiological study that has been conducted on psychosocial outcomes on adolescents and young persons in association with marijuana use.[3] There are birth cohort studies that provide the evidence of adverse effects.[11]

"Dried cannabis is not appropriate for patients who: Are under the age of 25; have a personal history or strong family history of psychosis; a current or past cannabis use disorder; an active substance use disorder; cardiovascular disease (angina, peripheral vascular disease, cerebrovascular disease, arrhythmias); respiratory disease; are pregnant, planning to become pregnant, or breast feeding. Dried cannabis should be authorized with caution in those patients who: Have a concurrent active mood or anxiety disorder; smoke tobacco; have risk factors for cardiovascular disease; are heavy users of alcohol or taking high doses of opioids or benzodiazepines or other sedating medications prescribed or available over-the-counter."[14] —The College of Family Physicians of Canada

The New Brunswick Medical Society on July 24, 2017, launched a public education campaign on marijuana health risks called *Legal Not Safe*.

Dr. Murphy-Kaulbeck, speaking for the organization, shared a concern for those using under the age of 25. The New Brunswick Medical Society had recommended the age of 25 as the earliest age for Canadians to access marijuana, raising it over the Federal Government's recommendation of the age of 18. The society subsequently lowered the suggested age to 21, deeming 25 as "unrealistic". [15]

In July of 2017 the New Brunswick Child and Youth Advocate issued an assessment of Bill C.45; calling for a prohibition of public smoking of marijuana, a prohibition of the smoking of marijuana in homes or vehicles where children are present and requested that the federal government conduct a Child Rights Impact Assessment to ensure the new legislation on marijuana legalization conformed with UN Rights of the Child Convention.[16]

4. Human Rights and Health

"Marijuana use is a victimless crime. Only if you do it on a desert island, quite alone, and nobody loves you."[1] —Peter Hitchens, *Stupid Arguments for Drug Legalisation Examined and Refuted*, 2017

Two divergent schools of public health theory emerged in the latter part of the 19th century, and both continue to influence modern global drug policy. The work of American Alfred Linedsmith formed the basis of harm reductionist theory. The work of Swedish psychiatrist Nils Bejerot took a prohibitionist stance of abstinence treatment, aligned with law enforcement who could address drug traffickers, as well as those who use drugs.

"Now, harm reduction, ideas inspired by Lindesmith, together with the anti-prohibition movement, and the International Harm Reduction Association states that 'harm reduction refers to policies, programs and practices that aim to reduce the harms associated with the use of psychoactive drugs in people unable or unwilling to stop'. The defining feature of this school of thought is the focus on the prevention of harm, rather than on the prevention of drug use itself, and the focus on people who continue to use drugs. The human rights they seek to protect are the rights of people to use or take illicit/ illegal/controlled drugs.

The rights of children to be protected from illicit drugs, as exemplified in *CRC Article 33* (*The Rights of the Child*) is being largely ignored in the drug policy debate inspired by the call for harm reduction which support the policy to tolerate illicit drug use while seeing to mitigate one or another of the myriad of the ill effects of drug use. Such policy is user-centered and not taking into consideration the best interest of the child. Such a policy is not child-friendly, only adult user-friendly."[2] —Datin Masni Mohd Ali, President of "BASMIDA" (national anti-drug association)

"In order to conform to the minimum human rights standards as set out in the *Convention on the Rights of the Child Article 33*, the national drug policy of countries that are parties to the *CRC* must be child-centered and not user-friendly."[3] —Josephine Baxter, Executive Director —Drug Free Australia

Concerns over drug use and resulting harm to children were raised in the 2007 report compiled by UNICEF Malaysia Commission, *Drug abuse & its impact on children and young people*: "Drug abuse by a family member will have a significant and enduring impact on the family dynamics and functioning. Families encounter great stress, conflict and anxiety as a consequence of trying to protect the family member from the dangers and harms associated with drugs, and to limit the damage arising from their behaviour towards the rest of the family.

A child's basic needs, diet and nutritional intake, health and schooling may become neglected if a parent is more preoccupied with drugs. A child may lose out on their childhood to adopt adult responsibilities having to provide both practical and emotional care for their parents who abuse drugs. A child may become the 'parent' if both parents are abusing drugs and unable to fulfil parenting roles and obligations. Older siblings may be expected to look after their younger brothers and sisters—to ensure they continue to go to school, to keep the home in order. A child faces a mix of anger, sadness, anxiety, shame, social isolation and loss as parents, siblings struggle with drug addiction. A child may develop drug problems as a result of being exposed to drug culture in the family."[4]

THE MARIJUANA CULTURE In Colorado, a marijuana drink is being sold as a punch available in *Pineapple Mango* and *Blue Raspberry*, with 151mg of THC per bottle.[5] The manufacturer's website states that the product is best used for "patients" with chronic pain of any kind or severity and its dosage is consistent, making it safe for consumers to medicate themselves with it throughout the day.[5] The company also manufactures marijuana chocolate bars. On one of the bars, at the bottom of the wrap in very fine lettering, is a warning in regards to not being suitable for children.[5] There are other products, including infused wine and beer, and an abundance of chocolate bars with 420mg THC content, with no visible warnings on the front packaging but rather enticing graphics, and phrases referring to the extreme potency offered.[6]

Headlines reveal that children are being hospitalized after ingesting marijuana edible products and suffering severe health complications.[7,8, 9,10,11,12] The reckless endangerment of children, and the corruption of minors are serious offenses and are applicable to exposing children to marijuana harms.

This includes leaving marijuana products in locations where young children can accidently get hold of them.

CHILD ENDANGERMENT   Five adolescents became ill after eating marijuana brownies that were sold to them by a seventeen year old.[13] Two of the students were unconsciousness when admitted to a Richmond, Virginia hospital and three other were treated for nausea and vomiting. The alleged marijuana seller was arrested on suspicion of selling drugs on a school campus as well as child endangerment.[13]

Seventy-five percent of all high school students in America have used addictive substances, including tobacco, alcohol, marijuana or cocaine, with one in five of them meeting the medical criteria for addiction (2011).[14]

A study sponsored by MetLife Foundation found a continued increase in marijuana use amongst adolescents since 2008.[15] "Heavy monthly use of marijuana (20 times or more in the past 30 days) has reached alarming levels. Nearly one out of every ten teens say that they used marijuana twenty times or more in the past month. This finding represented an 80% increase since 2008. The significant reduction of government funded prevention programs in the past few years may well be one factor for these increases in marijuana use," offered the researchers.

"In 2015, 27% of past-month high school users (more than 5% of all high school students) used (marijuana) daily or near-daily. Concerning age of first use, 41% of high school seniors who had ever used said they had first used by the age of 14 or before and another 43% had first used by the age of 16. Smoking was the most popular method of use with 87% of high school students stating it was their delivery method of choice."[16] —*Monitoring Health Concerns Related to Marijuana in Colorado* (2016)

School aged youth, who use marijuana products are reporting that they are having trouble stopping the use of these products.[17]

A CASA report found one in four American who began using any addictive substance before the age of 18 was addicted, compared to one in twenty-five Americans who started using at the age of twenty-one or older. [19] A 2004 report, also from CASA, reported that more teens were in substance abuse treatment for marijuana than for alcohol or all other illegal drugs combined.[18]

DRUG CONTROL "All one can reasonably expect from prohibition of any undesirable behavior is that it will substantially reduce the frequency and intensity of that behavior, to the net benefit of society."[20] —Harold Kalant, M.D. Ph.D. Toronto, Canada

LONG STANDING AGREEMENTS The first international drug conference was held in Shanghai in 1904. It was convened to discuss the global control of opium and other dangerous drugs. Co-ordinated international drug control began in earnest with the 1912 *International Opium Convention*, a treaty which placed restrictions on the movement of opium, a derivative of the poppy plant. The Egyptian and Turkish delegates to the 1912 conference requested that cannabis be included as a controlled substance.

"While opium was still the major consideration...there is, however, another product, which is at least as harmful as opium, if not more so, and which my government would be glad to see in the same category as the other narcotics already mentioned. I refer to hashish, the product of cannabis sativa. This substance and its derivatives work such havoc that the Egyptian government has for a long time past prohibited their introduction into the country. I cannot emphasize sufficiently the importance of including this product in the list of narcotics, the use of which is to be regulated by this conference."[21] —Dr. El Guindy, Egypt.

Additional drug control treaties were adopted by most countries: In 1961, the *Single Convention on Narcotic Drugs, The Convention on Psychotropic Substances* in 1971, and in 1988 the *United Nations Convention Against Illicit Traffic in Narcotic Drugs and Psychotropic Substances.*

After World War II, the international agreements on control of dangerous drugs become the responsibility of the United Nations. When the World Health Organization (WHO) was created in 1948, a Committee on Drug Dependence was created in an advisory capacity to the United Nations Commission on Narcotics. The committee concluded that in regards to marijuana "that use of the drug was dangerous from every point of view, whether physical, mental or social."[22]

Parties to the UN drug control conventions are required; "firstly to take all practicable measures for the prevention of the abuse of narcotic drugs or psychotropic substances. Secondly they should take steps for the early identification, treatment, education, aftercare, rehabilitation and social reintegration of the persons involved, who may have become dependent upon these substances."[23]

The Convention on The Rights of the Child Treaty was ratified, by the majority of United Nations member states in 1989 and it remains the most universally endorsed human rights treaty globally. *The Convention* sets out the basic human rights that children everywhere have in 54 articles and two optional protocols. There are a number of Articles within the CRC, which explicitly require Member States to focus their policies on how they will impact on current and future generations. The CRC is specific about the devastation caused by illicit drugs and the associated need for child protection.

Article 3: "In all actions concerning children, whether undertaken by public or private social welfare institutions, courts of law, administrative authorities or legislative bodies, the best interests of the child shall be a primary consideration."

Article 6: "Every child has the inherent right to life and that Member States shall ensure to the maximum extent possible the survival and development of the child."

Article 27: "Recognize the right of every child to a standard of living adequate for the child's physical, mental, spiritual, moral and social development."

Article 33: "States Parties shall take all appropriate measures, including legislative, administrative, social and educational measures, to protect children from the illicit use of narcotic drugs and psychotropic substances as defined in the relevant international treaties, and to prevent the use of children in the illicit production and trafficking of such substances."[24]

Three UN member state countries have not ratified the CRC, they are Somalia, South Sudan, and the United States. The United States is party to all three UN drug conventions. Canada is party to the three, as well as the *Convention on the Rights of the Child*.

HIDDEN HARMS OF DRUG USE "The factors most commonly associated with the occurrence of child abuse and neglect, and identified in families involved with child protection services, are domestic violence, parental substance abuse and parental mental health problems."[25] —Australian Institute of Family Studies (AIFS). In 2008, research compiled by the AIFS found that a substantial number of Australian children are living with adults routinely misusing alcohol and other drugs. The research showed that in cases of substantiated child abuse or neglect, 64% of parents experienced significant problems with substance and alcohol abuse. It is estimated, that 30% of abused or neglected children go on to maltreat children when they become adults.[26]

In the UK, the Advisory Council on the Misuse of Drugs (ACMD) issued a report in 2011 entitled *Hidden Harm*: Of parents with serious drug use problems, 37% of fathers and 64% of mothers remained with their children.[27]

In the United States, NIDA estimates the majority of all child abuse and neglect cases substantiated by child protective services involve some degree of substance abuse by the child's parents.[28] Most states in America, along with the District of Columbia, Guam, and the U.S Virgin Islands have laws within their child protection statutes that address the issue of substance abuse by parents. Individual state statures address prenatal drug exposure and the harm caused to children by exposure to illegal drug activity in their homes or environment. The information for each state is available through— the Child Welfare Information Gateway, Washington, DC, USA, and Department of Health and Human Services —Children's Bureau. The following are example excerpts:

Alaska Stat. 11.51.110: "A person commits the crime of endangering the welfare of a child in the second degree if the person, while caring for a child under age 10: Causes or allows the child to enter or remain in a dwelling or vehicle in which a controlled substance is stored in violation of chapter 11.71: Is impaired by an intoxicant, whether or not prescribed for the person, and there is no third person who is at least age 12 and not impaired by an intoxicant present to care for the child."[29]

Colorado Rev. Stat. 19-3-401(3) (b)-(c): " Court orders shall not be required in the following circumstances: When a newborn child is identified by a physician, registered nurse, licensed practical nurse, or physician's assistant engaged in the admission, care, or treatment of patients as being affected by substance abuse or demonstrating withdrawal symptoms resulting from prenatal drug exposure; when the newborn child is subject to an environment exposing the newborn child to a laboratory for manufacturing controlled substances."[30]

Arkansas Ann. Code 12-18-103(14) (B):"Neglect' shall include: Causing a child to be born with an illegal substance present in the child's bodily fluids or bodily substances as a result of the pregnant mother's knowingly using an illegal substance before the birth of the child....A test of the mother's bodily fluids or bodily substances may be used as evidence to establish neglect under this subdivision."[31]

HOME GROWN AND DANGEROUS Growing marijuana indoors poses serious health problems as it provides ideal conditions for the growth of toxic organisms. The three most dangerous strains of *aspergillus, fumigitus, flavus* and *niger* exist naturally on the marijuana plant. A deadly alfa-toxin can be associated with these strains, especially for individuals who are immune compromised. A 1996 study of 10,000 patients with invasive aspergillus, at Winchester Hospital in the UK, saw the cost per patient to treat or cure the disease rose to $63,000, for a total in costs of $633 million.[32]

Residents of Colorado who are age 21 or older are permitted to grow up to six marijuana plants in their homes for personal use. Plants have to be grown in a locked location, not in a garden or yard. Both counties and municipalities can pass stricter laws. If Bill C-45 passes into law as drafted, Canadians will also be allowed to grow marijuana plants in the home.

THE CURRENT WORLD VIEW Plans to legalize marijuana products, that are underway in various regions of North America, are being carried out in contradiction to the outcome of a Special Session (UNGASS), held in New York at the United Nations in April of 2016. At this meeting, world drug control partners recommitted to international cooperation in implement effective prevention, treatment and rehabilitation measures and acknowledged their ongoing responsibility to counter the world drug problem.

The cannabis legalization and regulation discussion paper of June 2016 reads: "Canada is party to the three major United Nations (UN) Conventions on narcotic drugs. In the context of the Convention, Canada is obliged to criminalize the production, sale and possession of cannabis for non-medical and non-scientific purposes. Legalization of marijuana is not in keeping with the expressed purposes of the drug convention."[33] On November 30, 2016, the Task Force wrote to the government: "While it is not part of the Task Force's mandate to make recommendations to the Government on how to address its international commitments, it is our view that Canada's proposal to legalize cannabis shares the objectives agreed to by member states in multilateral declarations, namely; to protect vulnerable citizens, particularly youth; to implement evidence-based policy; and to put public health, safety and welfare at the heart of a balanced approach to treaty implementation."[33]

In November of 2016, the Pontifical Academy of Sciences (PAS) held a meeting at the Vatican with international experts, led and inspired by Pope Francis and Queen Silvia of Sweden, to develop a global view of the current drug epidemic and recommendations to reverse the trend that imperils the elements of civil society: public health, safety and human progress. A statement was issued at the end of the meeting: "Millions of victims globally have succumbed to addiction. This is a contemporary version of slavery. It destroys autonomy and free will, a foreseeable outcome of using chemicals that artificially suppress and supplant natural brain reward systems in vulnerable people. Addiction especially threatens young people, as the vast majority of addictions can be traced to initiation during adolescence. This is a period of rapid brain development, with particular risk to the enduring harms of drug use. An essential priority is to protect the brains of children and youth, by discouraging use of all drugs.

The international epidemic is led by a globalized network of criminals and legal business interests, with children and youth as their primary targets. They have driven exponential growth of potent forms of cannabis, developed unclean highly addictive cocaine preparations, and created unregulated new psychoactive substances. Prescription drug diversion for non-medical misuse is rooted in different origins, but the risks of medication misuse can be as great or greater than illegal drugs.

We recommend the following actions to be taken: Support the three UN treaties governing licit and illicit drugs, which are signed by virtually every nation. These treaties permit medical use of drugs, with tight regulations to prevent diversion for non-medical use and which criminalize the nonmedical sale and use of these same chemicals. Governments have a moral and ethical responsibility to secure and defend the common good of their citizens. As trafficking of drugs imperils the health, security and the rule of law in nations, any compromise can be viewed as complicity.

Governments must unequivocally pursue drug trafficking at every level. They have a responsibility to denounce and criminalize corrupt banks, bankers and money launderers that profit from the drug trade, and thwart large scale and local drug trafficking. Governments must not engage in any public, private or covert agreements to gain financial support for political or personal reasons from drug traffickers or industries. Such agreements subvert the common good, trust, health and safety of their people, especially, their youth.

Instead, governments have a public health, legal and moral responsibility to confiscate the gains of these traffickers/industries and to use these proceeds to fund assistance programs for the victims, which include providing treatment, prevention and medical services, family support, as well as educational and employment opportunities. Governments should not use any ill-begotten gains from drug trafficking or sales to generate political messages, regulations or laws that foster use of abusable drugs and subvert public health and safety laws and regulations.

Reject drug legalization for recreational purposes as a hopeless, mindless strategy that would consign more people, especially the disadvantaged, youth, the poor and the mentally ill, to misery or even death while compromising civil society, social stability, equality, and the law.

Create a balanced drug strategy, coordinating public health and criminal justice systems to curtail supply, discourage drug use and promote recovery—as a more effective method to treat addiction than incarceration. The primary goal of addiction treatment is long-term care and recovery.

The foundations of this balanced strategy are fundamental human rights that include drug prevention and recovery among the world's diverse faith communities, with a special focus on the goal of protecting youth from drug sales and drug use, in accordance with *Article 33* of the *Convention on the Rights of the Child*. The prevention of addiction among youth (less than age 21) is a high priority, and achievable by rejecting the use of marijuana and other rewarding substances. The underlying reasons for this priority need to be conveyed to youth and their parents in collaboration with health, educational and local communities.

Educate the public with up-to-date scientific information on how drugs affect the brain, body and behavior, to clarify why legalization of marijuana and other drugs for recreational use is poor public policy, poor public health policy and poor legal policy. Harness religion to support substance abuse prevention and treatment. Drug use can devastate the soul and a loving relationship with God. Drug use in our communities tests our faith. The faithful have a precious opportunity to engage in preventing this tragic form of modern chemical slavery. For those now enslaved, they can confront the challenge of addiction and achieve their emancipation."[34]

ONE MILLION SIGNATURES SUPPORTING UN SANCTIONS ON NARCOTICS PRESENTED TODAY!! Dear Colleagues: On behalf of the Drug Prevention Network of the Americas and as a member of the Global Drug Prevention Network, I want to congratulate and commend Torgny Peterson and Malou Lindholm with the Hassela Nordic Network and Grainne Kenny with EURAD and all those who worked so hard to collect 1.3 million signatures for the 2003 Vienna Declaration, which was presented today, April 14, 2003, to Mr. Antonio Maria Costa, Executive Director, United Nations Office on Drugs and Crime and the UN Commission on Narcotic Drugs in Vienna. This is an impressive and powerful statement in support of responsible international anti-drug policies and against efforts by proponents of drug legalization to change and weaken UN Conventions on Drugs.... Together our voices will be heard!!! Best regards, Stephanie Haynes, Drug Prevention Network of the Americas, Global Drug Prevention Network.[35]

In the fall of 2017 the government of New Brunswick, Canada announced their intent to create a Crown corporation and revealed that they had signed memorandums of understanding with two licensed producers of marijuana in anticipation of the passing of legislation to legalize marijuana in all regions of Canada.

5. Drug Policy

THE OBAMA ADMINISTRATION AND MARIJUANA POLICY

The Office of National Drug Control Policy provided a statement, in regards to marijuana, on the government website under the presidency of Barack Obama: "Confusing messages being presented by popular culture, media, proponents of 'medical' marijuana, and political campaigns to legalize all marijuana use perpetuate the false notion that marijuana is harmless.... The Administration steadfastly opposes legalization of marijuana and other drugs because legalization would increase the availability and use of illicit drugs and pose significant and safety risks to all Americans particularly young people."[1]

On October 19, 2009, the Department of Justice issued a media statement: "Attorney General Eric Holder today announced formal guidelines for federal prosecutors in states that have enacted laws authorizing the use of marijuana for medical purposes. The guidelines make clear that the focus of federal resources should not be on individuals whose actions are in compliance with existing state laws, while underscoring that the Department will continue to prosecute people whose claims of compliance with state and local law conceal operations inconsistent with the terms, conditions, or purposes of those laws.

It will not be a priority to use federal resources to prosecute patients with serious illnesses or their care-givers who are complying with state laws on medical marijuana, but we will not tolerate drug traffickers who hide behind claims of compliance with state law to mask activities that are clearly illegal. This balanced policy formalizes a sensible approach that the Department has been following since January: effectively focus our resources on serious drug traffickers while taking into account state and local laws.

The guidelines set forth examples of conduct that would show when individuals are not in clear and unambiguous compliance with applicable state law and may indicate illegal drug trafficking activity of potential federal interest, including unlawful use of firearms, violence, sales to minors, money laundering, amounts of marijuana inconsistent with purported compliance with state or local law, marketing or excessive financial gains similarly inconsistent with state or local law, illegal possession or sale of other controlled substances, and ties to criminal enterprises."[2]

On August 29, 2013, the Justice Department announced: "Today, the U.S. Department of Justice announced an update to its federal marijuana enforcement policy in light of recent state ballot initiatives that legalize, under state law, the possession of small amounts of marijuana and provide for the regulation of marijuana production, processing, and sale. In a new memorandum outlining the policy, the Department makes clear that marijuana remains an illegal drug under the Controlled Substances Act and that federal prosecutors will continue to aggressively enforce this statute. To this end, the Department identifies eight enforcement areas that federal prosecutors should prioritize. These are the same enforcement priorities that have traditionally driven the Department's efforts in this area.

Outside of these enforcement priorities, however, the federal government has traditionally relied on state and local authorizes to address marijuana activity through enforcement of their own narcotics laws. This guidance continues that policy. For states such as Colorado and Washington that have enacted laws to authorize the production, distribution and possession of marijuana, the Department expects these states to establish strict regulatory schemes that protect the eight federal interests identified in the Department's guidance. These schemes must be tough in practice, not just on paper, and include strong, state-based enforcement efforts, backed by adequate funding. Based on assurances that those states will impose an appropriately strict regulatory system, the Department has informed the governors of both states that it is deferring its right to challenge their legalization laws at this time. But if any of the stated harms do materialize—either despite a strict regulatory scheme or because of the lack of one—federal prosecutors will act aggressively to bring individual prosecutions focused on federal enforcement priorities and the Department may challenge the regulatory scheme themselves in these states."[3] The memorandum, was sent out by Deputy Attorney General James M. Cole.

Eric Holder served as the Attorney General in the Obama administration from 2009 to 2015. In 2013, the Cole Memo signalled to federal officials not to prosecute marijuana businesses in legalized states, as long as they didn't violate certain provisions, such as not selling cannabis to minors or diverting product to the underground market or states without legalized cannabis.

Whether or not leading world health organizations are impactful in holding both the USA and Canada to long standing international treaties and conventions, that bar the legalization of marijuana for domestic markets, remains to be determined, or if sanctions are levied.

In 2015, Congress passed a law prohibiting the US Department of Justice from enforcing federal law in states with "medical marijuana".[4] This resulted in the Food and Drug Administration being prohibited from taking effective action in the "medical marijuana" states. The law was up for renewal on July 13, 2017.

Ahead of the July 13, 2017 vote, a letter with endorsements from a host of American drug prevention agencies, some led by individuals who had participated in the Parent Movement of the 1980s, was addressed to the chair-persons of the US House Appropriation Committee.[5] The letter was in response to the 2018 spending bill. The spending bill presented before the Appropriations Committee did not contain the medical marijuana rider that had been included and signed into law for the previous couple of years. It was anticipated that language from the previous *Rohrabacher-Farr Amendment* would be added to the 2018 spending bill. If included and passed, the Department of Justice would be precluded from being able to pursue violations of federal law by organizations involved in marijuana for medical purposes. The previous rider had also facilitated marijuana industry's ability to recruit investment funds and advance their agenda, it had also paved the way for them to make contributions to individuals running for political office.

5. Drug Policy

CANADA ON POT   Marijuana products for medical purposes were legalized in Canada by a judicial decision in 2001. The pot lobby were instrumental in effecting changes to Canadian law, in terms of marijuana access, production and distribution, as they stood as plaintiffs in numerous legal initiatives.

The Canadian government wrote to the Mayor of Vancouver on April 23, 2015, to express their official position on the municipal council's decision to provide a regulatory framework for illegal marijuana stores operating in the city of Vancouver: "While Canadian courts have required the government to allow access to marijuana when authorized by a physician, the law is clear that this must be done in a controlled fashion to protect public health and safety. In response to the courts, the government implemented the Marihuana for Medical Purposes Regulations (MMPR) in June 2013, with the aim of treating dried marijuana as much as possible like other narcotics used for medical purposes.... These regulations are clear and do not provide municipalities with the authority to legitimize the commercial sale of marijuana, which remains an illegal substance. Storefronts and dispensaries do not operate within a 'grey zone,' and the law is clear: they are illegal."[6] —Hon. Rona Ambrose PC MP (former) Minister of Health.

Canada saw a change in government in 2016, with the Conservative led government of Stephen Harper being replaced by the Liberals, under Justin Trudeau.

On March 26, 2017, the *CBC* announced they had learned from an unidentified source that the Canadian government would be introducing a marijuana legalization bill in the House of Commons in April 2017, with implementation by July 1, 2018.[7] The following day, the stocks of the licensed marijuana produced rose significantly. The source of the leaked information was not made public.

On April 10, 2017, The Royal Canadian Mounted Police (RCMP) told the *Canadian Press* that it was too early to know if the legalization of marijuana would affect the criminal involvement in the illicit marijuana market.[8] The federal Justice Minister Jody Wilson-Raybould, and other MPs along with the Prime Minister, had repeatedly stated that their new regulatory regime would "keep it out of the hands of children and the proceeds out of the hands of criminals."[9]

On April 13, 2017, the federal government of Canada held a media conference to discuss their marijuana plan. The president of Canada's first legal grow operation told the Canadian media that he thought the move was good from an industry perspective but a move that would be bad for society.[10] The grower said he agreed with the doctors and the police officials who wanted to see the minimum age at 21—even to 25 for higher potency product. This experienced Canadian grower also told the media that the push to legalization marijuana was "premature".[10]

Cannabis Canada, a licensed producer, issued a media statement on the news of impending legalization, calling the bill an important first step that "catapults" Canada into a global leadership position in the new industry sector.[11]

The Justice Minister stated; "the bill is permissive to the provinces and territories to reflect their specific factual situations."[12] One of the key factors that could determine the impact of legal access on the black market is the level of taxation that is placed on marijuana products. The federal government plans to leave taxation levels, and other details such as the final age for access, as well as distribution systems to the individual provinces.

5. Drug Policy

A *CBC* journalist asked the four Ministers of the Government attending the media briefing: "What if a province doesn't play ball?"[13] The federal government had allowed just 15 months to find a consensus with the provinces, which given the depth of this policy change has left them open to criticism as being overly ambitious. In June of 2017, a number of Canadian provincial governments announced that they might not be able to adequately address the legal, social and health challenges in time for the proposed implementation date of July 1, 2018.[14] The Minister of Justice for the Province of Manitoba relayed that he had raised the issue of an extension of implementation with the federal government.[14] The Prime Minister of Canada responded: "We gave everybody lots of time. We've been working for a long time with all the provinces, with the municipalities. It's time for us to move forward on this."[15] The Canadian Finance Minister took the position that for provinces that aren't ready in time for the "fixed date, the federal government would step in and oversee a mail-order sales program.[15]

On May 11, 2017, an MP in the House of Commons rose to ask Canadian Prime Minister how the government planned to end the long-standing international agreements that restricted the development of a legal marijuana retail market.[16] A member of the official opposition entered a petition opposing Bill C-45 into the House of Commons.[16]

STORMY WATERS AHEAD FOR AMERICA Representatives Dana Rohrabacher (CA), Earl Blumenauer (OR), Don Young (AK), and Jared Polis (CO) on February 16, 2017, launched the Congressional Cannabis Caucus. The newly formed caucus, a bi-partisan group of federal law makers, represents

Colorado, Oregon, California, and Alaska. On February 23, 2017, a media release was issued by the organization, outlining their disappointment over Sean Spicer's statement regarding "greater enforcement", and the possibility of a crackdown on the adult use of marijuana by the federal government.[17]

On February 23, 2017, White House Press Secretary Sean Spicer announced to the press: "I do believe you'll see greater enforcement."[19] He added that "it" will be a question for the Department of Justice.[19] California Lt. Gov. Gavin Newsom, a leading supporter of *Proposition 64*, sent a letter on February 24, 2017 to President Trump, urging him not to carry through with threats to launch a federal enforcement effort.[20] Amy Margolis, an attorney whose law firm represents clients who are involved with marijuana businesses told the *Los Angeles Times* that due to the maturity of the marijuana industry, if the federal government did start enforcement there could be legal challenges.[21]

In mid-May of 2017, statements made by the US Attorney General, Jeff Sessions raised concern within the marijuana lobby and industry as evidenced by their internet posts and chatter.[22] On May 12, the Attorney General addressed the Sergeants Benevolent Association of New York City and in his speech he made it clear that the Trump Administration was intent on returning to the enforcement of the law.[23]

"According to a report by the *New England Journal of Medicine*, the price of heroin is down, the availability is up and the purity is up. We intent to reverse that trend. So we are returning to the enforcement of the law was passed by Congress – plain and simple. If you are a drug trafficker, we will not look the other way. We will not be willfully blind to your conduct. We are talking about a kilogram of heroin—that is 10,000 doses, five kilograms of cocaine and 1,000 kilograms of marijuana. These are not low-level offenders. These are drug dealers. And you're going to prison."[23] —USA Attorney General Jeff Sessions

In July of 2017, US Attorney General Jeff Sessions wrote to the Governor of Colorado, after reviewing the 2016 Rocky Mountain High Intensity Drug Trafficking Area statement on the impact on marijuana legalization in the state. The Attorney General wrote in his letter that the report raised serious questions about the efficacy of the marijuana "regulatory structures" in Colorado. [24]

On March 16, 2017 pediatricians in the Colorado reported on the death of an 11 month old child from myocarditis after exposure to marijuana. The child with no known medical history, with normal development, with no trauma, was admitted to an ER with central nervous system depression, and unresponsive. He subsequently went into cardiac arrest and died.[25]

A lawyer was called as an expert witness before the Canadian House of Commons Standing Committee on Health on September 13th. 2017 to defend the legalization of marijuana in Canada. In support of Bill C. 45 he asked the panel of elected officials: "Where are the bodies?" There are those that deny the harm from marijuana and there are that propel this fallacy. This government witness was John Conroy and his travel to Ottawa was paid for by the taxpayers of Canada.[26]

6. Big Pots of Gold

Marijuana lobbyists were operational in the 1960's, but it would not be until the early 1990's that major financial players would contribute to, and energize, their efforts.

On December 2, 1996, Thomas A. Constantine, Administrator Drug Enforcement Administration of the United States Department of Justice, delivered the following statement before the Senate Committee on the Judiciary regarding, The California & Arizona Medical Drug Use Initiatives: "Mr. Chairman, Members of the Committee: I appreciate this opportunity to appear before the Committee today and discuss the issues surrounding the two recently-passed ballot initiatives in California and Arizona which, in essence, legalize the possession of marijuana, and in Arizona, all Schedule I drugs, such as heroin and LSD for medical purposes by 'seriously or terminally ill patients.'

Most Americans have not yet grasped the consequences of what happened last month in California and Arizona, and it is critical that Congress provide factual information about these initiatives. It is also critical that Americans understand that these legalization initiatives were not local, grass-roots efforts, but part of a well-orchestrated, well-financed national movement, not for the compassionate medical use of marijuana, but to legalize drugs. These efforts will have a profound impact on our children, as they struggle to grow up against the backdrop of increased drug use among young people.

Today we are faced with more questions than answers as we examine the impact of these initiatives. It is fair to say that both propositions were well-crafted and well-thought out, and their authors fully intended to mask their true agenda in the guise of drug 'medicalization,' while keeping the medical conditions for which controlled substances can be used extremely vague. The passage of these propositions raises important legal and law enforcement issues which we are currently assessing. But there are two very basic facts that have not changed: first, that the Clinton Administration is unequivocally opposed to the legalization of drugs, and second, that the Drug Enforcement Administration will continue to target and arrest the most significant drug traffickers operating domestically and internationally.

What the propositions do: Voters who supported *Proposition 215* in California were led to believe that this initiative would simply allow medical doctors to treat terminally ill and suffering patients with marijuana for the relief of pain symptoms. In reality, the proposition allows anyone who receives a doctor's 'recommendation' to possess and use marijuana for cancer, AIDs, glaucoma and 'any other illness for which marijuana provides relief.' It allows doctors to verbally 'recommend' marijuana use to minors, prisoners, and individuals in sensitive positions—simply anyone who claims to have a medical condition. The proposition, by extension, also allows individuals to smoke and cultivate marijuana openly, on the premise that marijuana has been recommended for the individual's 'medical condition.'

In Arizona, voters were asked to approve the *Drug Medicalization, Prevention and Control Act of 1996.* Packaged as a truth-in-sentencing and drug prevention measure, proponents masked the true agenda of *Proposition 200.* Buried within the proposition was a provision which allows a physician to prescribe controlled substances included in Schedule I to terminally ill patients and to seriously ill patients suffering pain.

The Arizona proposition is more restrictive than the California version in that a physician must cite a study confirming the proven medical benefits of a Schedule I drug and provide a written prescription which is kept in the patient's medical file, and the patient is required to obtain a written opinion from a second physician confirming that the prescription for the Schedule I substance is 'appropriate to treat a disease or to relieve the pain and suffering of a seriously ill patient or terminally ill patient.' However, the Arizona proposition also provided for other actions which erode effective, tough drug policies, including the release of prisoners 'previously convicted of personal possession or use of a controlled substance.'

Despite the differences between the two ballot initiatives, there is an indisputable similarity: both states now allow individuals to possess substances which have no legitimate medical use. Both California and Arizona, despite what the proponents claim, have taken the first steps towards the proponents' ultimate goal of legalizing drugs.

Who supported the proposition—*Proposition 215* in California and *Proposition 200* in Arizona were drafted, financed and supported by legalization proponents using the compassionate pain argument as a guise for their drug legalization agenda. Billionaire financier and legalization advocate, George Soros, provided hundreds of thousands of dollars in California alone to garner support for the proposition. In Arizona, Soros almost doubled his California donations, a significant portion of which were made through organizations, such as the Drug Policy Foundation, with which he is affiliated.

Other donors included representatives from the Progressive Corporation, the Men's Warehouse, and other pro-legalization groups. Proponents waged a sophisticated, misleading campaign which led voters to believe that the initiatives were simply limited to compassionate pain relief. Opponents of the propositions, including the American Cancer Society, the California Medical Association, the Glaucoma Research Foundation, the National Multiple Sclerosis Society, the California Narcotics Officers Association and many family groups concerned about the impact of drug legalization on the nation's children, were outspent and out-campaigned by the well-orchestrated effort to legalize drugs on a national basis. These individuals cynically used the suffering and illness of vulnerable people to further their own agenda.

Those of us who fought against the initiative, including General McCaffrey, myself, HHS Secretary Shalala and former Presidents Ford, Carter and Bush, found it extremely difficult to engage the media in California and Arizona and discuss the real issues underlying these propositions. Even the fact that 13,000 members of the International Association of Chiefs of Police, meeting in Phoenix, Arizona in late October, passed a resolution strongly opposing these initiatives, received little attention."[1]

The statement continues on to provide background details on the 1992 DEA position on the use of marijuana products for medical purposes and the agency's denial of the NORML petition to re-schedule the drug. The statement continues with implications for law enforcement: "I would like to discuss a few scenarios which raise questions and graphically illustrate the practical issues which face law enforcement in light of these developments. Can state and local law enforcement officers seize marijuana in California, and in Arizona, marijuana and other Schedule I drugs from individuals claiming to have received them as a result of a doctor's recommendation or prescription? Are these substances medicines under state law or contraband? Are police officers liable if they let individuals with marijuana, who claim a medical condition, drive off and later injure or kill someone? Are state and local officers able to detain individuals possessing Schedule I drugs, and call federal officials to come and arrest them on federal charges? How will the federal government meet the burdens of charging and prosecuting cases previously handled on a state level—without any additional resources and with already staggering workloads?

How will law enforcement officers respond to large marijuana plots when the owners claim that they are "caregivers" who must cultivate marijuana for their customers suffering from AIDS, cancer, or whatever medical conditions they identify? Can inmates in prison claim that they are suffering from a medical condition requiring treatment with Schedule I substances? Are prison officials obligated to allow the inmates to use these drugs? If so, how are prison officials in Arizona expected to maintain order and discipline with the inmates high on heroin, marijuana, LSD or other Schedule I drugs?

How will law enforcement handle prescriptions or recommendations from doctors or caregivers from other states, or from Mexico and Canada? These are serious questions which now face California and Arizona law enforcement officials on a daily basis. There are also significant issues which face the citizens of both states. Parents should ask how these propositions will impact on the safety of their children; will workplaces, including schools and transportation, maintain drug-free requirements? How will parents be assured that their child's Little League Coach or scoutmaster is not using drugs?

Perhaps the biggest question of all, however, is what impact the liberalization of drug policy will have on our children at a time when drug use has increased. The mixed messages we are sending will most likely have a terrible effect on parents' ability to provide unequivocal information about drugs to their young children.

What the Federal Government can do: The California and Arizona initiatives do nothing to change federal drug enforcement policy. The DEA will continue to target major drug traffickers, including major marijuana growers and distributors. We also can take both administrative and criminal actions against doctors who violate the terms of their DEA drug registrations that authorize them to prescribe controlled substances.

Doctors are registered with the DEA to prescribe only Schedule II-IV substances. Technically, those doctors who prescribe or recommend Schedule I substances are violating federal law. The licenses of over 900 physicians have either been surrendered or revoked in the last two years for fraudulent prescription practices.

The DEA is working with the Department of Justice and

the Office of National Drug Control Policy to ensure close coordination between the federal government, and state and local law enforcement agencies. We have met with officials from California and Arizona in an effort to ensure that they have the necessary support from the federal government, but there are still many issues to be worked out. Although there are no guarantees, the DEA is hopeful that continuing consultations with state and local officials will ensure that the citizens of both states will be protected from major drug traffickers and unscrupulous medical practitioners. In some cases, they will be one and the same.

Mr. Chairman, it is important for us to recognize that the proponents of drug legalization will not stop with California and Arizona. They intend to support and finance initiatives in many other states. Citizens of California can overturn this proposition in 1998 through another ballot initiative. It is possible for the Arizona legislature to overturn *Proposition 200* within a shorter period of time.

We should keep our attention focused on the next tier of states targeted by the legalizers, and should learn from the California and Arizona experiences. I firmly believe that the legalizers will pour millions of dollars into legalization campaigns, and will work diligently to disguise the legalization issue as a compassionate pain relief issue. However, we must continue to educate Americans about the true nature of the debate, and ensure that they have the facts necessary for them to make a sound decision.

It is instructional to look at what happened in Alaska after marijuana was decriminalized between 1975 and 1990. Marijuana abuse among teenagers doubled during that time period, and parents recognized the need to re-criminalize marijuana. In 1990, Alaskans voted to re- criminalize marijuana after a grass-roots effort educated voters in that state about the consequences of a liberalized drug policy. With marijuana use among 12–17 year olds dramatically increasing, and with surveys indicating that 35% of our children list drugs as their number one concern, we need to provide our next generation with the leadership necessary to reverse the current trends.

We need to put our energies and limited resources into reducing the demand for drugs, not legalizing them. I firmly believe that most Americans recognize how dangerous and counterproductive these propositions are, and with encouragement and a fair airing of the pros and cons of the issue, they will stand up to the legalizers and their millions of dollars."[1]

FUNDS POURED IN The *Follow the Money* website is operated by the nonpartisan, non-profit, National Institute on Money in State Politics. The website provides campaign-donor information and other information from government disclosure, with the aim of providing accountable democracy.

The three parties that are shown to have given the most to pro-marijuana campaigns were, The Marijuana Policy Project, Drug Policy Alliance, and former Progressive Insurance Chairman Peter B. Lewis.[2] The data shows that a number of pro-drug lobbying groups operating in Washington D.C. and New York, along with wealthy individuals, invested millions of dollars to influence drug policy in the United States.[2]

Follow the Money.com compiled the contributions made to legalization efforts between 2004 and 2014, and found that supporters of legalization were persistently assisted by wealthy donors, many of whom lived out of the state where legalization was on a ballot initiative.[2] For the period under review, the researchers found that legalization forces were ahead in terms of funds raised by $28.2 million; with $29,981,310 in funds raised to support legalization with opponents with $1,777.588.[2] Sixty three percent of the money supporting state ballot initiatives for marijuana came from out-of-state donors. Over ninety percent of the funds raised, to support the legalization of marijuana in Colorado in 2012, was out of state money.[2]

Arnold Trebach set up The Drug Policy Foundation (DPF) in 1987. The DPF organizes educational lobby sessions and trains for drug legalization advocates in the United States and from Canada, the Netherlands, Switzerland, Germany, England, Australia and Israel. The Lindesmith Center, a drug policy think-tank, with the aim of being the world's leading drug policy reform organization, was established in 1994. It was the first US project for George Soros' Open Society Institute.[2] The two organizations merged to form The Drug Policy Alliance in 2000. Drug Policy Alliance total revenues for the fiscal year ending May 20, 2012, amounted to roughly $48.7 million, not including the income or expenses for the related advocacy and political arm of the Drug Policy Alliance (Drug Policy Action).[3]

The Marijuana Policy Project Foundation was founded in 1996, and helps to support the efforts of the Marijuana Policy Project (MPP). For the fiscal year ending December 12, 2012, total revenue was $3,533,657.00, not including the income or expenses for the related advocacy and political arm of the Marijuana Policy Project Foundation.[4] Between 2003 and 2016 the Marijuana Policy Project hired 168 lobbyists, operating in many jurisdictions.[4]

6. Big Pots of Gold

It is estimated that Peter Lewis had spent between 40 million and 60 million dollars to fund the cause of legalization since the 1980s.[2]

An Inside Look At The Biggest Drug Reformer In The Country: George Soros, ran in *Forbes* on October 2, 2014. Chloe Sorvino reported the donations by George Soros, through his charities to drug reforms, were in the amount of approximately $200 million since 1994.[5] The largest portion of the funds reportedly went to the non-profit Drug Policy Alliance.[5]

"The pro-legalization movement hasn't come from a groundswell of the people. A great deal of its funding and fraud has been perpetrated by George Soros and then promoted by celebrities. The truth is under attack, and it's an absolutely dangerous direction for this country to be going in."[6] —John Walters, director of the White House Office of National Drug Control Policy under George W. Bush

A legal marijuana market in North America is potentially worth vast sums of money, however this could all change if sales and industrial expansion are impeded by legal challenges, including those coming from the federal level, or from the public sector, in the form of class action law suits advanced by injured parties.

The present US federal government could see major changes to national drug policy enforcement and pose difficulties for states that have moved on legalizing marijuana products for any purpose.

THE AMBITIOUS MARIJUANA INDUSTRIALISTS "We don't invest in U.S. companies that touch the product directly," said Mr. (Brendan) Kennedy, Privateer Holdings Inc. CEO.[7]

"They are not so shy about Canada," wrote Brian Hutchinson, in an interview with Kennedy; *Medical marijuana production in Canada set for dramatic change*, for the *National Post*.[7] Privateer Holdings owns Leafly.com, Marley Natural, and Canadian based Tilray. Lafitte Ventures Ltd. is Privateers' Canadian subsidiary and has a marijuana license from the Government of Canada.

"For us it is about reaching the biggest market with the most professional brand."[8] —Michael Blue, Privateer Holdings Inc. C.F.O.

"You know it's a massive industry now and you know it will only grow as further legalization takes place and you know if you look globally, you know it is a hundred and fifty billion dollar industry. That is the only reason you know why we jumped into the space."[8] —Brendan Kennedy

According to the American research firm CB Insights, in 2014 funding in the marijuana industry grew upwards of 941.5%, adding over $104 million to the sector over the previous year.[9] Privateer Holdings Inc., of Seattle, was reported to have raised the largest amount, followed by the Chicago-based PharmaCann group and Leafline Labs of Minnesota.[9]

Reuters on January 9, 2015, reported that Peter Thiel's venture capital firm, The Founders Fund, had confirmed that it would be taking a minority stake in Privateer Holdings.[9] "We're fine with investing in business with regulatory ambiguity, because we believe that regulation follows public sentiment," said Geoff Lewis, a partner in The Founders Fund.[10]

Privateer Holdings, in partnership with the descendants of Bob Marley are creating a multinational cannabis brand called *Marley Natural*. Named after the famed musician Bob Marley, it is reported that investors raised $50 million for the launch of *Marley Naturals* in November of 2014.[11]

"This is what the end of prohibition look like....By contrast *Marley Natural* will look like a modern consumer product, cleanly packaged and marketed with the help of the same agency that branded *New Balance* and *Starbucks Coffee*,"[11] Brendan Kennedy told *NBC News*.

Leafly placed the first consumer cannabis advertisement in *The New York Times*, on August 2, 2014, in response to New York Governor Andrew Cuomo recent signing of the *Compassionate Care Act* into law, on July 7, 2014. The ads tagline reads; "Just Say Know, Congratulations on the Compassionate Care Act, NY! The first step in benefitting from cannabis is making informed choices. From learning the right products and strains for you, to finding trusted clinics and dispensaries nearby, we'll be there to help. A Privateer Holdings Company. Ian chose an indica cannabis strain to relieve his MS symptoms. While fighting cancer, Molly preferred sativa cannabis."[12]

"Our advertisement in *The New York Times* is a responsible, mainstream message that elevates the conversation about cannabis in the US," said Brendan Kennedy, speaking with the media on August 4, 2014.[12] Whether the ad "elevates" the conversation or is rather an attempt to direct public opinion through marketing tactics is debatable. It remains an open question as to whether the ad serves to undermine existing federal laws that prohibit the use of marijuana for any purpose in all regions of the United States. The USA FDA, does not support the use of marijuana as medicine or permit the advertising of controlled substances.

Data from Follow the Money shows Privateer Holdings Inc.

hired fourteen lobbyists in New York and Washington for the years; 2013, 2014, and 2015.

In July 2011, the United States FDA reaffirmed marijuana as a Schedule 1 substance. In April of 2015, a Federal Court Judge in the State of California upheld the constitutionality of a 1970 federal law, which classified cannabis as a dangerous drug. U.S. District Judge Kimberly J. Mueller, announcing her decision, said she could not lightly overturn a law passed by Congress.[13] The hearing marked the first time in decades that a judge examined the classification of marijuana under the 1970 Controlled Substances Act.

The government's expert witness was Dr. Bertha Madras, a former deputy director for demand reduction in the White House Office of National Drug Control Policy. Judge Mueller acknowledged that a majority of qualified scientists believe marijuana has no current medical use. Mueller said the existence of principled disagreements, among reputable scientists and practitioners, regarding the potential benefits and detrimental effects of marijuana showed that Congress' dangerous-drug classifications was not arbitrary or irrational.[14] To be an approved medicine the FDA requires certain criteria must be fulfilled. One of the criteria is that the drug must be accepted by well-qualified experts.

"Marijuana is not an approved medication, does not come in specific dosages or concentrations, and cannot be prescribed. However, there is anecdotal evidence which suggests that some component or components of marijuana may be useful for patients with chronic pain, side-effects of chemotherapy and with varying symptoms secondary to HIV infection. In no case have any double-blind placebo-controlled trials demonstrated objectively measurable benefits from the whole plant, either for these purposes or for any medical application."[15] —Stuart Gitlow, M.D., M.P.H. M.B.A.

A second criteria that must be met prior to FDA approval is that the scientific evidence of efficacy must be widely available. "The evidence for approval of medical conditions in state ballot and legislative initiatives did not conform to rigorous, objective clinical trials nor was it widely available for scrutiny."[15] —Dr. Bertha Madras

"Cannabinoids have many roles in the central and peripheral nervous systems and the autonomic nervous system. That's why we have so many cannabinoid receptors. So smoking dope will inevitably activate some of these receptors with various outcomes, including mild analgesia. Of course the risk/adverse effects far outweigh the potential benefits or therapeutic value of smoking doobies or eating MJ brownies." —Ray Baker M.D. F.C.M.P., F.A.S.M.[15]

The delegates at the 2013 Interim Meeting of the American Medical Association (AMA) voted to pass a resolution on marijuana, explicitly opposing marijuana legalization: "Our AMA believes that (1) cannabis is a dangerous drug and as such is a public health concern; (2) sale of cannabis should not be legalized."[16]

"The AMA today reiterated the widely held scientific view that marijuana is dangerous and should not be legalized," said Dr. Stuart Gitlow, Chair-Elect of the AMA Council on Science and Health.[16] He added: "We can only hope that the public will listen to science—not 'Big Marijuana' interests who stand to gain millions of dollars from increased addiction rates."

The American Psychiatric Association position on

marijuana for medical purposes reads: "No current scientific evidence that marijuana is in any way beneficial for treatment of any psychiatric disorder. In contrast, current evidence supports, at minimum, a strong association of cannabis use with the onset of psychiatric disorders. Adolescents are particularly vulnerable to harm, given the effects of cannabis on neurological development."[17]

Michael D. Privitera, M.D., (former) president of the American Epilepsy Society and director of the Epilepsy Center at the University of Cincinnati Neuroscience Institute, wrote to a Pennsylvania legislator: "The families and children moving to Colorado are receiving unregulated, highly variable artisanal preparations of cannabis oil prescribed, in most cases, by physicians with no training in pediatrics, neurology, or epilepsy. As a result, the epilepsy specialists in Colorado have been at the bedside of children having severe dystonic reactions and other movement disorders, developmental regression, intractable vomiting and worsening seizures that can be so severe they have to put the child into a coma to get the seizures to stop. Because these products are unregulated, it is impossible to know if these dangerous adverse reactions are due to the CBD or because of contaminants found in these artisanal preparations. The Colorado team has also seen families who have gone into significant debt, paying hundreds of dollars a month for oils that do not appear to work for the vast majority. For all these reasons, not a single pediatric neurologist in Colorado recommends the use of artisanal cannabis preparations."[18]

In the United States, as of 2017, marijuana for non-medical use had been legalized by eight state governments as well as

The District of Columbia. Twenty nine states have authorized medi-pot.

In August of 2014, Kevin Sabet, Ph.D. with Smart Approaches to Marijuana, along with representatives from Colorado SAM, and concerned health professionals called on *The Denver Post* newspaper and Leafly to stop unfounded medical claims being broadcast about the benefits of their products.[19]

On August 25, 2014, Bob Doyle, on behalf of Colorado SAM, sent a letter to Brendan Kennedy of Privateer Holdings and of Leafly.com and copied members of the medical community: "We are writing to express serious concern regarding information Leafly.com makes available through *The Cannabist*, the online marijuana section of *The Denver Post*. The site's recommendations from Leafly state marijuana strains "treat" mental illnesses, including attention deficit/hyperactivity disorder (ADHA), bipolar disorder, depression, and post-traumatic stress disorder (PTSD).

In light of the serious potential impact of your recommendations, including possible delay in medical treatment for serious and potentially life threatening mental illnesses, and the potential worsening of those illnesses by the marijuana you recommend, we request that you release the data upon which these recommendations for dispensing the specific marijuana strains as a treatment for bipolar disorder, PTSD, ADHD, and depression are based. For each strain, we request to know the recommended dosage, duration, the THC and CBD content, whether you're recommending they be used with or without FDA approved medical or behavioral treatment for the condition, what contraindications are known, and whether other physical or mental health issues should preclude certain people from using the strain."[20]

In 2017, the *Leafly* website listed *Suicide Girl* as an available strain.[21] The recipe for this marijuana product was described as a cross of *Poison OG* with *Girl Scout Cookies*.[21] Highlights for the strain included its utilization in combating anxiety, depression and minor pain.[22] The claims included; "the beauty" and "potency" of the product, and that it delivers "hearty" mid-level sedation in the body, along with a "sizzling buzz to the brain".[22] Access to information on various strains and where to purchase on the *Leafly* website is without any restrictions. The *Leafly* website is a portal that provides the marijuana consumer with a list of products and where they are available. They are an American operation but their listings include marijuana companies across Canada. It is worth spending time on this site to understand the scope of this entity.[22]

"The claims frequently made by zealous users for the superior merits of one strain or another of cannabis for the treatment of different symptoms or diseases have no basis in scientific research, and can be disregarded by the physician."[23]
—Harold Kalant, M.D, Ph.D.

7. Prevention

SETTLING THE DEBATE OVER PORTUGAL A 2009 Cato Institute (USA) report, determined that drug use had not increased in Portugal under decriminalization.[1] The report was discussed in an article; *Drugs in Portugal: Did Decriminalization Work?*, *Time.com*, (2009).[2]

In January of 2017, Nathaniel Erskine-Smith, an MP in the government of Canada, told the *CBC* in Toronto, Ontario, that the changes in Portugal to decriminalize small possession and the use of all drugs, led to a decrease in teen drug use, drug overdoses and deaths, and criminal penalties dropped by 60%. Erskine-Smith has publically supported the decriminalization of all drugs.[3]

Five Myths about Legalized Marijuana, written by Doug Fine appeared in the *Washington Post*: "(In) Portugal...youth drug use rates fell after all drugs were legalized there in 2001."[4]

On June 10, 2013, Kevin Sabet, Ph.D., responded to the *Washington Post* column: "OK. A few things: First, Portugal never legalized any drugs. In 2001, they made law what was basically already in practice (there and in most other European countries) by not criminalizing personal drug use. Now, they refer all drug users to panels of social workers who determine the next course of action (dismissal, treatment referral, etc.). Also in 2001, Portugal increased its provision of treatment and prevention.

The result of these laws? It's difficult to say, since a number of other relevant changes took place in addition to this (relatively minor) change in the law. *The European Monitoring Centre for Drugs* and Drug *Addiction (EMCDDA)*, long considered the authority on drug statistics in Europe, compiled statistics showing an increase in lifetime prevalence rates for the use of cannabis, cocaine, amphetamines, ecstasy and LSD between 2001 and 2011. Those figures apply to the general population of Portugal, ages 15 to 64 years of age.

The European School Survey Project on Alcohol and Other Drugs (ESPAD) survey of 15- and 16-year-olds shows an overall increase in the prevalence of marijuana use between 1999 and 2011, although there was an initial dip in use rates. Past-month prevalence for marijuana in that age group went from 5% in 1999, to 3% in 2003, to 6% in 2007, and finally up 9% in 2011. *EMCDDA* concluded that the most recent *ESPAD* study corroborates the findings of the (UN World Health Organization) study; showing increasing consumption of illicit substances (in Portugal) since 2006. 'Besides the unjustified attribution of a causal effect to the change in policy, (Doug) Fine largely based his assertion on "lifetime prevalence" statistics, which do not tell us anything around recent use. His analysis also stopped at 2007, when we have more recent data from ESPAD and EMCDDA that shows increased use from 2001 to 2011."[5]

THE DUTCH DRUG EXPERIMENT In 1976, the sale and possession of up to a maximum of 30g of marijuana was decriminalized in Holland. With this move to more permissive drug policies, use rates nearly tripled between 1984 and 1996, rising from 15% to 44% among 18-20 year aged Dutch youth.[6]

In 2004, the average level of THC in home grown Dutch marijuana was 20.4%. Marijuana use and mental health became such an issue that in the Netherlands, cannabis with more than 15% THC was reclassified. The high potency marijuana is not allowed to be sold in Dutch weed-selling coffee shops.

Seventy percent of all Dutch towns have adopted zero tolerance policies toward cannabis cafes. From 2011 onward, tourists were banned from obtaining marijuana from any of the remaining marijuana coffee shops in Holland. Pot tourism had created many problems for the local residents and business owners.[6]

On December 31, 2017, the oldest cannabis coffee shop closed. The reason stated was the close proximity to a school.[7]

"The feeling of the Dutch people is that they have enough from drugs, criminality and brutality. However they haven't got the tools, the 'know-how' and belief that the drug problem can be solved. Politicians, mayors and others from the drugs industry are the one who set the agenda. The consequences of the disastrously liberal drug policy, Dutch drugs policy is a fiasco."[8] —Renée Besseling, *Parents a Natural Preventive Against Drugs, The Dutch experience*

The Dutch government accepted a controlled drug trade, regulated under the principals of harm reductionism, but in practise developed the Dutch drug industry of today. Holland is the only country, other than Canada, to issue export licenses for the selling of medi-pot.

THE AMERICAN POT ERA Between 1955 and 1965 the rate in the USA for marijuana product use was between 1–2% of the population.[9] The *Gallop Poll* of 1967, conducted by a national survey of college students, found a 5% lifetime use of marijuana products. In 1969 the rate was found to be 22% for both college age students and 17–18 year olds. Further surveying conducted in 1969 by Gallop, found only 1% of adults aged 50 and older had ever tried marijuana. In 1970, Gallop polling of college students found 43% with lifetime use, 39% with past year use, and 28% reported past month use.[8] In 1971, 51% of college students reported lifetime use, past year use reached 41%, and past month use rose to 30%.[9] In 1971 6% of 12–13 year olds had ever tried marijuana.[9] Of those reporting using, 2% of adults and 4% of youth reported using it more than once a day.[9] By 1972, 5% of 12–15 year olds, 11% of 16–18 year olds, and 8% of 18–22 year olds reported they were using every day.[9]

Just Say No, ran from the 1980s into the early 1990s. The widely publicized slogan was created by the First Lady Nancy Reagan, during her husband President Ronald Reagan's first term as President of the United States. The campaign was based on the work of Professor Richard I Evans, and was supported by The Girl Scouts of America, Kiwanis Club International and the National Federation of Parents for a Drug Free Youth, along with others. Five thousand *Just Say No* clubs were part of the campaign to educate American children to reject illicit drugs. The drug issue made national news broadcasts and the US Congress in 1986 passed anti-drug legislation backed by $1.7 billion in financing.[10]

Seventy percent of young people in a 1985 survey stated they abstained from marijuana products out of fear of the consequential physical or psychological damage, 40% abstained because of the law and 60% abstained out of concern over parental disapproval.[10] In 1969, just under half of Americans viewed drug use as a serious community problem but by 1986, 56% of Americans thought the government was not spending enough. In 1995, 65% of Americans viewed drug use as a 'serious problem' for the country. By the early 1990s, the decline reversed and new survey results showed an increase in the number of 17–18 year olds using across all prevalence categories. Between 1992 and 1994, past month use for 17–18 year olds had increased by 60%. Past month use by 13–14 year olds showed a 100% increase in the two year period, and for 15–16 year olds the increase was 95%.[10]

The current generation of North American youth are using marijuana products in numbers not seen since the 1970s. Three differences with the pot "fad" of the 1970s and 1980s and the current pot heyday, is the arrival of the marijuana industry, the introduction of higher potency products, and the reach of the heavily funded, politically connected, marijuana lobby.

DECLINING POPULARITY OF MARIJUANA "Societies tend to react against drugs slowly, and the reaction usually comes just after the popularity of drugs has peaked."[11] —Dr. David Musto

In 2004, the British government downgraded marijuana to Class C from Class B. In 2008 the average THC content of 80% of the UK skunk market had risen to 16% potency. In 2009, the drug was prudently restored to Class B.[12]

"If only we had known then what we can reveal today. Record numbers of teenagers are requiring drug treatment as a result of smoking skunk, the highly potent cannabis strain that is 25 times stronger than resin sold a decade ago —An Apology."[13] The editorial was published by *The Independent* on March 18, 2007 with

a follow up the following week. "*The Independent on Sunday* has changed its view because of the growing weight of evidence that cannabis contributes to mental illness. As we made clear last week, what was a law-enforcement argument about priorities in 1997 has become, in 2007, a medical debate about mental health."[14] —*The Independent*

In 2009, a new direction was taken with UK drug strategy with a focus on drug prevention, and reducing demand. An extract from the "*UK Drug Strategy*" reads: "Specific and measurable strategies are in place that will aim to; break inter-generational paths to dependency by supporting vulnerable families; provide good quality education and advice so that young people and their parents are provided with information to actively resist substance misuse; intervene early with young people and young adults; consistently enforce effective criminal sanctions to deter drug use; and support people to recover….A national programme will focus on helping to turn around the lives of families with multiple problems. Education and information for all. All young people need high quality drug and alcohol education so they have a thorough knowledge of their effects and harms and have the skills and confidence to choose not to use drugs and alcohol. Schools have a clear role to play in preventing drug and alcohol misuse as part of their pastoral responsibilities to pupils. Some family-focused interventions have the best evidence of preventing substance misuse amongst young people. Intensive family interventions are highly cost effective with every £1 million invested achieving £2.5 million in savings to local authorities and the state."[15]

In August of 2015 a petition to make the production, sale and use of cannabis legal was submitted to the British

Government: "Legalising cannabis could bring in £900m in taxes every year, save £400m on policing cannabis and create over 10,000 new jobs. A substance that is safer than alcohol, and has many uses. It is believed to have been used by humans for over 4000 years, being made illegal in the UK in 1925."[16]

The UK Government responded: "Substantial evidence shows cannabis is a harmful drug that can damage health. There are no plans to legalise cannabis as it would not address the harm to individuals and communities. The latest evidence from the independent Advisory Council on the Misuse of Drugs is that the use of cannabis is a significant public health issue ('Cannabis Classification and Public Health', 2008).

Cannabis can unquestionably cause harm to individuals and society. Legalisation of cannabis would not eliminate the crime committed by the illicit trade, nor would it address the harms associated with drug dependence and the misery that this can cause to families. Legalisation would also send the wrong message to the vast majority of people who do not take drugs, especially young and vulnerable people, with the potential grave risk of increased misuse of drugs.

Despite the potential opportunity offered by legalisation to raise revenue through taxation, there would be costs in relation to administrative, compliance and law enforcement activities, as well as the wider costs of drug prevention and health services. The UK's approach on drugs remains clear: we must prevent drug use in our communities; help dependent individuals through treatment and wider recovery support; while ensuring law enforcement protects society by stopping the supply and tackling the organised crime that is associated with the drugs trade. The Government will build on the *Drugs Strategy* by continuing to take a balanced and coherent approach to address the evolving challenges posed. There are positive signs that the Government's approach is working: there has been a long term downward trend in drug use over the last decade, and more people are recovering from their dependency now than in 2009/10. The number of adults, aged 16–59 using cannabis in the last year in England and Wales, has declined over the last decade from 9.6% to 6.7%, with cannabis use amongst young adults aged 16–24 and young people aged 11–15 following a similar pattern."[17]

According to a report from Europe's drug monitoring agency, the *EMCDDA*, the number of Britons aged 15 to 34 using cannabis has almost halved in little more than a decade, with statistics from the year 2000 establishing that almost 20% of the country's young adults were using marijuana, whereas the figures, from 2013, indicate that rate had dropped to just above 10%.[18]

PSYCHOSIS AND MARIJUANA USE COSTS "For example, cannabis use in the UK increased four-fold between 1970 and 2002, and increased 18 fold in the under 18s. They estimated that the new cases of schizophrenia would increase by 29% in men between 1990 and 2010. In fact, it later found that the annual new cases of schizophrenia and psychoses increased from 49 per 100,000 in 1990 up to 77 per 100,000 in 1999, an increase of 58% over three years. In general, studies found that psychosis occurs 2 to 8 years after a significant amount of cannabis use, and that the risk of psychosis is higher when cannabis use starts at an earlier age."[19] —T.H. Moore and colleagues, *The Lancet Psychiatry*

"Any future increases in cannabis-associated new cases of schizophrenia would add to the current high rate in Canada. M.J. Dealberto at Queen's University in Ontario, found that the rate of new cases of schizophrenia in Canada is about 26 per 100,000 per year, considerably higher than the countries outside Canada which average about 12 new cases per 100,000 per year. (Quebec is even higher at 40.)

In addition, such an increase in new schizophrenia cases would need to be matched by significant increases in psychiatric hospital budgets and in community-based housing and welfare. For example, Ontario's two major psychiatric centers (Ontario Shores Centre for Mental Health Sciences in Whitby, and the Centre for Addiction and Mental Health in Toronto) have a combined annual budget of about 400 million dollars, with approximately half assigned for schizophrenia.

Across Canada, such budgets would need major increases. Considering that Ontario, for example, receives about 1,100 million dollars each year for tobacco taxes, a cannabis tax might cover the increased needs of the psychiatric hospitals and the community housing. While the majority of cannabis users would not develop schizophrenia, the wider use of cannabis would lead not only to more hospitalizations of the new cases of schizophrenia, but also to an increased confrontation of psychotically disturbed young men with police."[20]
—Dr. Philip Seeman, University of Toronto, Canada

A white paper, issued by Smart Approaches to Marijuana Vermont, authored by Christine L. Miller Ph.D. and Dean Whitlock, determined that the legalization of marijuana would lead to an increase in the number of people with mental illness, including schizophrenia.[21] By the author's estimates this would increase the tax burden on the state of Vermont by between $4.9 million and $11.1 million dollars.[21] A media release announcing the findings reads: "Similar studies on poor health outcomes from tobacco and alcohol use moved society to try and limit rather than increase their presence in our culture, without waiting for the exact mechanism of caution to be fully understood."[22]

A new type of marijuana product was reported by *Drug Watch International* on February 25, 2008 called *Budder* and was identified as having between 82–99.6% pure THC.[23] In the 1960s and 1970s marijuana was a balance of low THC and CBD, as it exists in its natural non-altered state. "Skunk use alone was responsible for 24% of adults presenting with first-episode psychosis to the psychiatric services in South London."[23] —*The Mail Online*, 2015

In May of 2017, a study was released establishing that marijuana-related emergency visits by youth, between the ages of 13–21 in Colorado, between January 2005 and June 2015, more than quadrupled with the legalization of marijuana.[24] Sixty six percent of the 3,443 marijuana-related visits during the study period were related to symptoms of mental illness. Approximately half of the young people attending an emergency room for a marijuana-related medical issue also tested positive for other drugs, including ethanol, amphetamines, benzodiazepines, opiates and cocaine as the most common found substances.[24]

"In 2010, 7.3 percent of all persons admitted to publicly funded treatment facilities were aged 12 to 17."[25] —Center for Behavioral Health Statistics and Quality.

"On an average day, 881,684 U.S. teenagers aged 12 to 17 smoked cigarettes. On an average day 646,707 adolescents smoked marijuana and 457,672 drank alcohol."[26]
—SAMHSA (2013)

REVERSING COURSE In 1995, under pressure from both the international drug prevention community and from within Holland, the Dutch Government reduced the amount of marijuana permitted to be carried to 5g. from the 1976 limit of 30g. The formal policy of non-enforcement of the possession and sale of a limited amount of marijuana remains in effect.

8. Change Has To Come

THE CONNECTION WITH DAMAGE Of the millions upon millions of people worldwide who have used marijuana products, many may not have detected or acknowledged harm as a result. Marijuana has been widely promoted as a benign product, explained as both a harmless herb and powerful wonder cure. Beyond the temporary experience of intoxication or neurological impairment many users may not know of the long-lasting physiological ramifications that follow use.

One potential risk is the negative health outcomes to the future offspring of people who use these products. Of the various risk factors linked with the use of marijuana products, the risk of generational DNA damage—or "chromosomal shattering", is perhaps the most compelling argument for continuing strict restrictions.

WARNING "In my twenty years of research on human cells, I have never found any other drug, including heroin, which comes close to the DNA damage caused by marijuana."[1] —Dr. Akira Miroshima, authority on cytogenetics and formerly of Columbia University College of Physicians and Surgeons.

Health Canada requires all licensed sellers of marijuana

for medical purposes to distribute Health Canada's consumer information, along with marijuana consumer orders. The information is provided in; *Government of Canada Consumer Information: Cannabis (Marihuana, marijuana)*.[2] It reads: "The courts in Canada have ruled that the federal government must provide reasonable access to a legal source of marijuana for medical purposes....

Cannabis is not an approved therapeutic product and the provision of this information should not be interpreted as an endorsement of the use of cannabis for therapeutic purposes, or of marijuana generally, by Health Canada. This leaflet is designed by Health Canada for patients authorized to possess cannabis for medical purposes. It is based on the document *Information for Health Care Professionals: (marihuana, marijuana) and the Cannabinoids*, and is a summary only—it will not provide you with all the facts about cannabis for medical purposes. Contact your health care practitioner if you have any questions....

SERIOUS WARNINGS AND PRECAUTIONS: Keep any fresh or dried marijuana and cannabis oil out of reach of children. Cannabis (marihuana, marijuana) contains hundreds of substances, some of which can affect the proper functioning of the brain and central nervous system. The use of this product involves risks to health, some of which may not be known or fully understood. Studies supporting the safety and efficacy of cannabis for therapeutic purposes are limited and do not meet the standard required by the Food and Drug Regulations for marketed drugs in Canada. Smoking cannabis is not recommended. Do not smoke or vaporize cannabis in the presence of children.

Using cannabis or any cannabis product can impair your concentration, your ability to think and make decisions, and your reaction time and coordination. This can affect your motor skills, including your ability to drive. It can also increase anxiety and cause panic attacks, and in some cases paranoia and hallucinations. Cognitive impairment may be greatly increased when cannabis is consumed along with alcohol or other drugs which affect the activity of the nervous system (e.g. opioids, sleeping pills, other psychoactive drugs).

WHEN THE PRODUCT SHOULD NOT BE USED: Cannabis should not be used if you: Are under the age of 25/ are allergic to any cannabinoid or to smoke/ have serious liver, kidney/ heart or lung disease/have a personal or family history of serious mental disorders such as schizophrenia / psychosis / depression / or bipolar disorder/are pregnant/are planning to get pregnant/or are breast-feeding/are a man who wishes to start a family/have a history of alcohol or drug abuse or substance dependence."[2]

THE THALIDOMIDE PARALLEL The risks are so severe for thalidomide, in terms of use in pregnancy that a special protocol that educates, evaluates, mitigates and monitors has been made obligatory. Thalidomide (Contergan®) was developed by a German company, Chemie Gruenenthal, in 1954 and approved for the consumer market in 1957. It was available as an over-the-counter drug for the relief of "anxiety, insomnia, gastritis, and tension" and later it was used to alleviate nausea and to help with morning sickness in pregnancy.

Thalidomide was present in at least 46 countries under a variety of brand names and was available in "sample tablet form" in Canada by 1959 and licensed for prescription on December 2, 1961. Although thalidomide was withdrawn from the market in West Germany and the UK by December 2, 1961, it remained legally available in Canada until March of 1962.[3] It was still available in some Canadian pharmacies as late as the middle of May of 1962.[3] Canadian authorities had permitted the drug onto the Canadian market when many warnings were already available.

An association was being made in 1958 of phocomelia (limb malformation) in babies of mothers using thalidomide.[4] A trial conducted in Germany against Gruenenthal, for causing intentional and negligent bodily injury and death, began in 1968 ending in 1970 with a claim of insufficient evidence.[4] Later, the victims and Gruenenthal settled the case for 100 million dollars.[5]

In 1962, the American pharmaceutical laws were increased by the *Kefauver-Harris Drug Amendment* of 1962 and proof for the therapeutic efficiency through suitable and controlled studies would be required for any government approved medication.[6] According to paragraph 25 of the Contergan foundation law, every 2 years a new report is required to determine if further development of these regulations are necessary to insure patient safety.

In 1987 the War Amputations of Canada established The Thalidomide Task Force, to seek compensation for Canadian-born thalidomide victims from the government of Canada and then in 1991, the Ministry of National Health and Welfare (the current Health Canada) awarded Canadian-born thalidomide survivors a small lump-sum payment. In 2015 the Canadian government agreed on a settlement of $180 million dollars to 100 survivors of thalidomide drug exposure and damage.

Through Rona Ambrose, in her capacity as the Health Minister at the time of the negotiations, an attempt was made to involve the drug companies related to the thalidomide issue in the survivor's settlement agreement. Negotiations with the drug companies failed. The Canadian taxpayer alone paid to amend the survivors by way of monetary award.[7]

Thalidomide continues to be sold under the brand name of Immunoprin®, among others in a REMS program. It is an immunomodulatory drug and today, it is used mainly as a treatment of certain cancers (multiple myeloma) and leprosy.

MARIJUANA RISKS Risks demonstrated in the scientific literature include chromosomal damage.[8] When exposure occurs in utero, there is an association with many congenital abnormalities including cardiac septal defects, anotia, anophthalmos, and gastroschisis.[8] Marijuana use can disrupt foetal growth and the development of organs and limbs and may result in mutagenic alterations in DNA.[8] Cannabis has also been associated with foetal abnormalities in many studies including low birth weight, foetal growth restriction, preterm birth spontaneous miscarriage, spina bifida and others. Phocomelia has been shown in testing in a similar preclinical model (hamster) to that which revealed the teratogenicity of thalidomide.[8, 9]

"THC has the ability to interfere with the first stages in the formation of the brain of the fetus; this event occurs two weeks after conception. Exposure to today's high potency marijuana in early pregnancy is associated with anencephaly, a devastating birth defect in which infants are born with large parts of the brain or skull missing."[8] —Reece, A.S. and Hulse G.K, Australia

Warnings and the contraindications for use of marijuana for medical purposes by specific populations and in association with identified conditions, have been publicized by the Federal Government of Canada and the Federal Government of the United States of America through their respective health agencies. [2, 9, 10, 11]

PROTECTIVE MEASURES NEEDED   In the spring of 2017, the Toronto Transit Authority was granted the right through a judicial ruling to conduct random drug and alcohol tests on their employed drivers of subways, buses and streetcars. Employees within the Commission, who hold safety-related roles in maintenance, control or the executive, would also be required to submit on demand to substance testing. This move to random testing was taken after a bus-driver rear-ended another vehicle, killing a female passenger in 2011.[12]

Once again policy changes followed the witnessing of damage, again in response to the death of an individual rather than through foresight. Such damage avoidable, preventable, if only protective measures had been put in place earlier.

The evidence that thalidomide, and tobacco products were harmful was known to the manufacturers and distributors before the populous acknowledged these dangers. To date, there continue to be legal repercussions to those who knowingly place the public at risk. Since both the United States and Canadian government health agencies are fully aware of the marijuana harms, these government must not be complicit in risking citizens health, but rather must mitigate any and all such risk to current and future generations.

As the stewards of human and financial resources, it is

critical that governments protect the public from potential irreversible harm and itself from litigation risk by harmed individuals knowing that, in the context of marijuana use, harm is not only possible but probable.

All marijuana products, including marijuana for medical purposes, fit the prerequisites for a REMS or Revaid Program.[13, 14] For regions that have adopted legal access to marijuana products implementing a strict drug dispensing and monitoring protocol; no less arduous than that used for the delivery of drugs such as thalidomide are called for out of concern for patient safety and human rights.

9. Drugged and Driving

"Drug use is considered by many to be a victimless 'crime', yet those killed or injured by drug-impaired drivers demonstrate the simplicity of this argument." —Ed Wood President, DUID Victim Voices

There is substantial evidence that recent marijuana use by a driver doubles their risk of a motor vehicle crash.[1] When combined with a little amount of alcohol, marijuana drivers are at eight fold the risk of a crash compared to a normal drug-alcohol-free driver.[2]

Given that a typical marijuana cigarette in Colorado contains approximately 0.5 grams of marijuana, and todays' THC content in marijuana ranges from 12-23%; a typical joint contains 60-115 mg THC; six to ten individuals, who are less-than weekly users, sharing one such joint, would find their ability to drive meaningfully impaired. The standard "legal" serving size for a marijuana edible is 10mg in the state of Colorado.[3,4]

2016 evidence statements, from The Colorado Department of Public Health and Environment, included the following: "We found SUBSTANTIAL evidence that marijuana users who use less-than-weekly, there is meaningful driving impairment with a whole blood THC of 2-5 ng/mL. We found

SUBSTANTIAL evidence that for marijuana users who use less-than-weekly, smoking more than 10mg THC (or part of a currently available marijuana cigarette) is likely to meaningfully impair driving ability.

We found SUBSTANTIAL evidence that for marijuana users who use less-than-weekly, orally ingested 10mg or more of THC is likely to meaningfully impair driving ability. We found SUBSTANTIAL evidence that delaying driving for at least 6 hours after smoking less than 18mg THC allows THC-induced impairment to resolve or nearly resolve for users who use less-than-weekly. We found SUBSTANTIAL evidence that delaying driving at least 8 hours after oral ingestion of less than 18mg THC allows THC-induced impairment to resolve or nearly resolve for users who use less-than-weekly."[4]

The 2015 study by R. Hartman, et al., published in *Drug and Alcohol Dependence*, showed that using a simulated driving system and participants who were infrequent marijuana users that, following smoking marijuana, a 13.1 ng/mL THC blood level at the time of driving produced the same lateral movement (weaving) as 0.08 BAC.[5] The study also showed that at 1.4 hours after driving, the mean level ranged from 3.9 to 5.7 ng/mL THC and after 2.3 hours from driving the mean ranged from 2.2—3.2 ng/mL THC depending on the THC concentration in the joint (2.9% or 6.7% THC, respectively).[5] A THC level of 5 ng/mL at the time of driving plus a low blood alcohol concentration (0.05) produced the same amount of road weaving at 0.08 BAC.[5]

A further study in 2016, *Accident Analysis and Prevention*, also conducted by R. Hartman, et. al., shows that a DRE law enforcement officers may accurately (with 96.7% accuracy rate) identify a marijuana-positive driver if the driver has two or more failures on the Standard Field Sobriety Test.[6] Standardized road sobriety testing is the gold standard of detection of alcohol impairment of individuals capable of being tested. (Those seriously injured in an accident for obvious reasons are eliminated from such testing.) The four tests for marijuana impairment include the finger to nose test, one legged stand test, walk and turn test, and eyelid tremors during a modified Rhomberg test.[6] Roadside testing devices, including visual testing and breath tests for marijuana, could be specifically useful in providing early drug identification. Currently, a THC saliva test is available for early detection. Breath tests are in development.

Tanya Guevarra and her newborn son were both killed, by a driver who confessed to driving under the influence of marijuana. The driver tested positive for 4ng/mL of THC (drawn at an unknown time after driving).[7]

In December of 2015, 24 year old Lakeisha Holloway drove her car onto a sidewalk in Las Vegas Nevada USA, killing one person and injuring dozens.[8] Holloway's blood levels for active marijuana was 3.5 ng/mL and the metabolite was 23.6 ng/mL, higher than the threshold established in Nevada of 2 ng/mL THC, to convict a person for driving under the influence of marijuana. Holloway was charged with murder, leaving the scene of an accident, and child endangerment as Holloway's three year-old daughter was in the vehicle at the time of the crash.[8]

2013 data, roadside screening and post-mortem reports indicate that driving after drug use is now more prevalent among young people than driving after drinking.[9] In 2015, more drivers killed in auto crashes tested positive for drugs than alcohol, according to an updated report from the Governors'

Highway Safety Association and the Foundation for Advancing Alcohol Responsibility.[10] Drugs were present in 43% of fatally injured drivers with known test results, appearing more frequently than alcohol. Of the 57% of fatalities tested, 35.6% were positive for marijuana.

"A number of the youth believed that cannabis is safe and makes people better drivers by increasing their focus. Drunk driving was seen as being much more dangerous than driving under the influence of cannabis. In contrast, others felt that using cannabis while driving is dangerous and constitutes impaired driving. However, even those opposed to using cannabis and driving stated that it is not as dangerous as drunk driving."[11] —CCSA (2014) Driving drugged in Canada has increased in recent years despite a decline in alcohol impaired driving.[11]

Marijuana specifically impacts the crucial driving skill of double attention, particularly for the occasional user.

A Canadian national study of fatally injured drivers reported that between 2000 and 2010 a total of 20,485 drivers died in motor vehicle crashes.[12] Of the drivers who died within six hours of the crash, 33.7% tested positive for one or more psychoactive drugs during this period. Nearly 17% (16.6%) of all tested cases were positive for cannabis, accounting for almost half (45.4%) of all drug-positive cases.[12]

Juristat indicates in Canada for 2013, there were 78,391 police-reported incidents of impaired driving, of which only 1,984, or 3%, involved drug-impaired driving for the entire country.[13] Given the rates of use in Canada of marijuana products and the data now available from both Washington and Colorado, it would appear as though there is vast under-reporting or detection of Canadian drivers who are operating a vehicle impaired from the use of marijuana.[14]

In 1999, an 18-year-old was among five teenagers killed outside Perth, Ontario, Canada in a collision involving a young driver who had used marijuana before getting into the vehicle. "Where we are today with drugs is where we were 25 years ago with alcohol...That's how far behind the curve we are," said the father of one of the deceased teens in an interview with the *CBC*.[15]

Thirty-four years ago, neuroscientist Dr. Goodman wrote: "In a recent Canadian study among 15-19 year olds involved in fatal accidents, 44% were driving with discernable levels of THC in their blood. A third time I suspected society might have an overly generous and forgiving attitude towards marijuana was at the time of the government's campaign against drunk driving. Police efforts were increased to get the drunken drivers off the road. The campaign was certainly worthwhile. Yet marijuana is an intoxicant too."[16]

In 1910, New York was the first state to adopt drunk-driving laws—all other states would follow. Early DUI laws specified, that a driver could not be intoxicated while operating a motor vehicle. Intoxication was not definitively defined until the 1930s, when it was determined that a driver, with a determined blood alcohol concentration (BAC), could be presumed to be inebriated. Erased was the argument that a person, who was impaired by alcohol, could defend themselves with an argument of "bad" driving. In 1938, 0.15% became the first commonly-used legal limit BAC.

As a result of efforts by groups, such as Mothers against Drunk Driving (MADD) and Students against Drunk Driving

(SADD), changes came to DUI laws, including the setting of drinking age. The age of twenty-one was set for all states, under the passing of the Federal Uniform Drinking Age of 1984. In the 1980s, enforcing drunk driving laws became a larger priority for law enforcement, due in large part to the work of advocate groups and the survivors of victims of roadside homicides who fought for change.

Individual states continue to have flexibility and control over alcohol policy development and enforcement. The original 0.15 percent, set in the 1930's would come to be lowered and then reduced further to 0.08%, with zero tolerance laws put in place by some states. In 2004, all 50 states adopted the .08 BAC standard and implementation of the *per se* laws. Such laws establish that if an individual is tested and their BAC is .08 or over, no additional evidence of intoxication is required, the individual is considered intoxicated under the law. This nationwide adoption was aided by the US Congress limiting Federal highway funding to only those states that adopted the law.

"Driving is a privilege, not a right." —Phillip Drum, Pharm.D.

All states define alcohol DUI *per se* with laboratory tests, that prove impairment by a blood or breath alcohol level greater than .08 gm/dl for adults and greater than zero (or .02 gm/dl) for minors. Laboratory tests are routinely performed for all suspected alcohol DUI cases. Only 17 states define DUI drug (DUID) *per se* by objective laboratory tests. Three additional states have established permissible limits for marijuana's active THC in drivers, but these limits are a poor substitute for comprehensive drug *per se* laws. All other states use more difficult, costly, and subjective means to prove DUID on a case-by-case basis, with highly variable results.

Rosemary Tempel, R.N, B.S.N., B.C, C.Q.I.A. was 56 years old at the time she was driving to work at Virginia Mason Hospital in Seattle, WA. Speeding in the center turn lane, traveling in the opposite direction while under the influence of marijuana, Timothy Durden directed his Jeep directly into Rosemary's car. Durden's car catapulted over her car—crushing her and breaking her neck, then lost the two front wheels and tumbled down the busy road resulting in an 8 car pile-up. Upon up righting Durden's vehicle, a Seattle police detective saw marijuana and multiple business cards to Seattle's Herbal Health Care Center marijuana dispensary fall from Durden's vehicle. Durden volunteered to have his blood drawn 3 hours and 13 minutes after the incident. It was found to have 3.2 ng/ml THC.

During a pre-trial hearing on October 28, 2013, Judge Monica Benton threw out the marijuana blood evidence and thus the vehicular homicide (DUI) charge, stating she did not believe the Seattle PD Drug Recognition Expert's (DRE) testimony. That testimony was under oath and had written corroborating evidence. His driving without auto insurance at the time of the incident, previous possession of controlled substances, and selling cocaine and marijuana to an undercover officer were all withheld from the jury. Judge Benton had previous experience with Durden. She had earlier permitted Durden to continue his use of marijuana while on probation for a domestic violence charge, which was performed under the influence of marijuana and alcohol. On December 13, 2013, Timothy Durden was sentenced to 4.5 years following a jury conviction of vehicular homicide (reckless) + vehicular assault. Durden was released after serving 35 months.[17]

1997–2017: TWENTY YEARS TO GET IT RIGHT *Prop 64* states in section 34019 (c): "The Controller shall next disburse the sum of three million dollars ($3,000,000.00) annually to the Department of the California Highway Patrol beginning fiscal year 2018-2019 until fiscal year 2022-2023 to establish and adopt protocols to determine whether a driver is operating a vehicle while impaired, including impairment by the use of marijuana or marijuana products, and to establish and adopt protocols setting forth best practices to assist law enforcement agencies. The department may hire personnel to establish the protocols specified in this subdivision. In addition, the department may make grants to public and private research institutions for the purpose of developing technology for determining when a driver is operating a vehicle while impaired, including impairment by the use of marijuana or marijuana products."[18]

The California Highway Patrol (CHP) has been well funded since the *Compassionate Use Act* was approved in 1996 by the California voters. The CHP has had 20 years to establish and adopt protocols for a marijuana impaired driver and has failed to do so.

Based on the 2014 NHTSA's FARS data, at a minimum there are 0.8 marijuana positive driving deaths in California per day.[19] Based on analysis by A. Crancer and P. Drum, changing from a medical-marijuana state to a recreational marijuana state will lead to an increase in marijuana positive driving fatalities to 1.2 per day; based on what has transpired in Colorado, Washington, Oregon and Alaska.[19] There have been 1,338 marijuana-positive driving deaths of Californians from 2011 to 2015.[20]

In the 2013 U.S. FARS data base, only 62.6 % of driving deaths were tested for drugs other than alcohol.[21] Marijuana has been the second most common substance (after alcohol) since 2006 found in automobile deaths in California.[22] Based on the FARS 2015 data base, less than 25% of driving deaths in California were blood tested for drugs.[23] The actual number of deaths from marijuana driving may be vastly under-estimated.

Rates of driving fatalities in 2014 with the driver having marijuana in their blood for the State of Washington was 30.9%, Alaska 30.5%, Oregon 21.7%, and Colorado 20%.[24,25,26] All of these states have adult legal access to marijuana products. The average rate of a marijuana-positive driving fatality for non-legal marijuana states was 13.9%.[27] Legalized marijuana states (both medical and recreational) have a 28.5% higher marijuana driving fatality rate than non-legalized marijuana states.[27]

In 2014, driving deaths data shows marijuana-positive drivers were statistically more apt to have been speeding at the time of the crash, compared to no alcohol/no drug drivers (33% marijuana vs 24% no drugs/alcohol).[28] Marijuana's affect upon a driver includes the inability to stay in a lane (weaving), slower reaction time, a decreased ability to drive correctly, reduced attention—unable to respond to signals and sounds, and altered speed perception.[29] R. Hartman, et al, in a paper published in Clinical Chemistry (2013), showed these effects may last for up to 24 to 48 hours depending on the person.[29]

"It has been established that most alcohol fatalities (34.3%) occur in the early morning hours (10 pm—1:59 am) following bars closing on Friday, Saturday and Sunday.[30] This is true for alcohol positive fatal crashes in Washington in 2015. Fridays accounted for 19.2% of all driving fatalities for the week, Saturday (20.2%) and Sunday (28.3%). The time after the end of a normal work day (4 pm—7:59 pm) is the highest percent (28.4%) of fatal marijuana positive crashes during a day. Unlike alcohol, the incidence of day of the week of marijuana consumption is not concentrated around any day or group of days. There is a slight increase, but not statistically significant, in marijuana crashes occurring on Saturdays (19.3%) versus an average of 14.3% for equivalent daily usage.[30]

Marijuana use is combined with alcohol (BAC 0.01+) in 53.3% of marijuana driving fatality cases. Contrary to popular belief and urban myth, marijuana drivers in fatal crashes do speed and do so about as much as drivers who are DUI and about twice the percentage of all WA drivers in fatal crashes. The combination of alcohol plus marijuana positive driving fatalities peak from 6 pm to 9:59 pm."[30] —Cramer and Drum (2016)

Mixing marijuana and alcohol, even at low dosage is dangerous and places drivers and their passengers at risk. Alcohol causes a faster absorption of THC, slower elimination and can lead to a combined central nervous system effect than if marijuana was used on its own.

SETTING THE RECORD STRAIGHT ON TOXICOLOGY REPORT
"The state toxicologist of the Washington State Patrol released data showing that the percentage of driving cases testing positive for THC through blood tests jumped dramatically in the first four months of 2015 over previous years: 2009—18.2%, 2010 -19.4%, 2011-20.2%, 2012-18.6%, 2013-24.9%, 2014-28%, 2015-33% (limited January through April for 2015). Licensed recreational marijuana businesses opened in Washington in July 2014. Following a year and a half of sales, the marijuana driving fatality percentage has nearly reached alcohol driving fatalities for 2014 and 2015. The state toxicologist, Dr. Fiona Couper,

of the State patrol's laboratory reported in 2014 that virtually all 2013 blood samples were monitored for drugs, in addition to alcohol. Interesting, despite the testing for both alcohol and drugs when tests are performed on drivers in fatal crashes, the actual percentage of blood tests for alcohol and marijuana has been on the decline over 2014 and 2015. There has been a statistically significant reduction in alcohol blood testing from 64% in 2013 to only 52.2 % being tested in 2015, and for marijuana from 62.5% to 50.8% during the same time period. At the same time, there has been a statistically significant increase by 33% (from 592 to 788) in the number of total drivers in fatal crashes in WA."[31, 32] —Crancer and Drum (2016)

Historically, drug tests were not often performed if blood-alcohol levels came back at 0.10% or higher, thus underestimating the true occurrence of marijuana and other drugged driving in the past. The average cost of a blood drug test ranges from $150.00-$250.00.[33] The average 2 hour time between an automobile crash and blood draw, allows THC in the blood from smoked marijuana to decline by 90% or more, frequently below the level of detection (1 ng/ml THC), even for someone who was smoking at the time of the crash.[34]

In 2013, the WA state toxicologist changed the level of detection for THC from 1 ng/ml to 2 ng/ml.[35] This statistically lowered the number of marijuana positive individuals in 2013. In 2014, the WA state toxicologist reduced the THC limit back down to 1 ng/ml. There was a 32% increase in marijuana fatal drivers from 2013 (66 deaths) to 2014 (88 deaths) after only 6 months of recreational dispensaries being open in 2014.[36]

Colorado traffic deaths, with THC found in the driver, has doubled from 2009 (commercialization for medical marijuana) to 2014 (legalization for non-medical use).[37] There was an 87% increase in drivers testing positive for THC who were involved in fatal crashes in Colorado between 2013 and 2015. In 2015 of the 115 marijuana related traffic deaths 75 were drivers, 20 were passengers, 17 were pedestrians and 3 were cyclists.[38] Based on the 2010 US Department of Transportation estimate per driving fatality ($1.4 million per fatality) with a modest 2-4% increase in costs per year, the cost of the 115 documented THC-positive driving fatalities that occurred in 2015 in Colorado and not taking into consideration the cost of assaults, that caused bodily harm but not death; the total cost amounts to $184 million to the state.[39] The breakdown of costs by percentile; property damage 31%, market productivity 24%, congestion 12%, medical 10%, household productivity 8%, legal 5%, workplace 2% and insurance 8%.[39]

Measuring the loss to society against the Colorado marijuana tax revenue from the sale of marijuana for medical and non-medical use for Fiscal Year 2015 was an estimated $125.5 million.[40] The Colorado taxpayer was left with approximately with a loss of $58.5 million, not to mention all of the other social costs from marijuana—emergency room visits, hospitalizations for exposure, skin grafting for BHO explosions, addiction, and life-long educational losses in the children expelled from schools for marijuana use, injury on job costs, along with other costs.

Bryan Tanner was smoking marijuana, while driving, with his 4-year old daughter in the car at the time. He drove off the highway and crashed the vehicle. His child was seriously injured. A blood test confirmed he was marijuana impaired at the time of the crash.[41]

The driver in a single car crash in Brown Deer that took the life of a 3-year-old girl faced charges in her death. The 35 year old driver admitted to drinking and smoking marijuana before the crash, which also involved excessive speed. Lee admitted to smoking marijuana two or three hours before the crash and drinking a half bottle of liquor and two beers.[42]

Luther Stoudemire 18, Kassidy Clark 16, and Jenna Farley 14, lost their lives when the car they were riding in left the road, and hit a tree. The 17 year-old driver allegedly told officers he had smoked marijuana before the crash.[43]

Josiah Alves, 7, died in the front seat of his father's car in 2012. The father was on marijuana when he crashed the vehicle. A Snohomish Washington County Superior Court Judge sentenced John Alves to 15 months in prison. Vehicular homicide is not considered a violent offense. Prosecutors did not allege that Alves was driving under the influence of drugs. The father man would have faced up to 8 1/2 years in prison if he had been convicted of driving under the influence at the time of the crash. State toxicologists reported that Alves tested at twice the legal limit for THC.[44]

A spokesperson for State Farm, commented on the company's 2017 survey on attitudes on driving and the use of marijuana products on Canadian radio: "Just about 50 per cent believe that smoking marijuana and diving does not impact their ability to do so, so, we found that alarming. That's a five per cent increase on average over the same question we asked Canadians last year."[45]

In July of 2017, the Canadian media reported on an announcement by the federal government of a budget of $1.9 million to create a public education commercial to address young persons and driving drugged.[46] The media reported that the government was also putting out calls, seeking an agency to create the campaign.[46] With less than ago year to go for the target start date for implementation of legal access for Canadians 18 years of age and older it is questioned why they have waited so long before addressing this critical issue.

On mid September of 2017 the Canadian trucking industry called for zero tolerance polices for professional drivers. A legal expert told the Canadian media that such a position could face challenges under existing employment law and human rights. [47]

10. Colorado

"In November 2000, Colorado voters passed *Amendment 20* which permitted a qualifying patient and/or caregiver of a patient to possess up to 2 ounces of marijuana and grow 6 marijuana plants for medical purposes. *Amendment 20* provided identification cards for individuals with a doctor's recommendation to use marijuana for a debilitating medical condition.

From 2001–2008, there were 5,993 patient applications received and 55% of those designated a primary caregiver. During that time, the average was three patients per caregiver and there were no retail medical marijuana 'dispensaries'.

The dynamics surrounding medical marijuana in Colorado changed substantially after 2008. A Denver District Judge in late 2007, ruled against the five-patient-to-one-caregiver ratio, overturning the previous order. This opened the door for caregivers to claim an unlimited number of patients for whom they were providing and growing marijuana. This decision expanded the parameters, however very few initially began operating medical marijuana commercial operations (dispensaries) in fear of prosecution, particularly from the federal government.

The judge's ruling, and caregivers expanding their patient base, created significant problems for local prosecutors seeking a conviction for marijuana distribution by caregivers. Many jurisdictions ceased or limited filing such types of cases.

At a press conference in Santa Ana, California on February 25, 2009, the U.S. Attorney General was asked whether raids in California on medical marijuana dispensaries would continue. He responded "No" and referenced the President's campaign promise related to medical marijuana. In mid-March 2009, the U.S. Attorney General clarified the position saying that the Department of Justice enforcement policy would be restricted to traffickers who falsely masqueraded as medical dispensaries and used medical marijuana laws as a shield.

Beginning in the spring of 2009, Colorado experienced an explosion to over 20,000 new medical marijuana patient applications and the emergence of over 250 medical marijuana dispensaries (allowed to operate as "caregivers").

One dispensary owner claimed to be a primary caregiver to 1,200 patients. Government took little or no action against these commercial operations. In July 2009, the Colorado Board of Health, after hearings, failed to reinstate the five-patients-to-one-caregiver rule. On October 19, 2009, U.S. Deputy Attorney General David Ogden provided guidelines for U.S. Attorneys in states that enacted medical marijuana laws. The memo advised: 'Not focus federal resources in your state on individuals whose actions are in clear and unambiguous compliance with existing state law providing for the medical use of marijuana.'

By the end of 2009, new patient applications jumped from around 6,000 for the first seven years to an additional 38,000 in just one year. Actual cardholders went from 4,800 in 2008 to 41,000 in 2009. By mid-2010, there were over 900 unlicensed marijuana dispensaries identified by law enforcement.

In 2010, law enforcement sought legislation to ban dispensaries and reinstate the one-to-five ratio of caregiver to patient as the model. However, in 2010 the Colorado Legislature passed HB-1284 which legalized medical marijuana centers (dispensaries), marijuana cultivation operations, and manufacturers for marijuana edible products. By 2012, there were 532 licensed dispensaries in Colorado and over 108,000 registered patients, 94 percent of who qualified for a card because of severe pain.

In 2012, Colorado voters passed *Amendment 64*, which legalized marijuana for recreational use in private space but banned it in public space, including restaurants, bars. *Amendment 64* permits marijuana retail stores, marijuana cultivation sites, marijuana edible factories and marijuana testing sites."[1] — Rocky Mountain HIDTA Office of National Drug Control Policy USA.

Surge in Children Accidentally Eating Marijuana-Laced Foods: Relaxed Colorado Drug Laws Behind Trend. Science Daily: "A new study shows that the relaxation of marijuana laws in Colorado has caused a significant spike in the number of young children treated for accidentally eating marijuana-laced cookies, candies, brownies and beverages."[2]

Children's hospitalizations related to marijuana after legalization include: the death of an 11-month-old baby and nine children who had symptoms so serious that they ended up in the intensive care unit of Colorado Children's Hospital. Two children needed breathing tubes.[3]

Seventy-four percent of adolescents in a Denver substance abuse treatment program had used someone else's medical marijuana approximately 50 times or more.[4]

The Retail Marijuana Public Health Advisory Committee's report of January 2015: *Monitoring Health Concerns Related to Marijuana Use in Colorado 2014* states: "Though medical marijuana has been legal in Colorado since 2000, it was largely viewed as an individual doctor/patient decision outside the scope of public health policy. However, the legalization of retail (non-medical) marijuana and the potential for greater availability of marijuana in the community, prompted a closer look at potential health impacts on the population at large. In addition, this report presents data from a onetime survey of women, infants and children clients conducted by Tri-County Health Department in 2014 to assess marijuana-use and behaviors. Unfortunately, prior to 2014, there was no funding source for adding questions about marijuana to Colorado's major public health surveys including the *Behavioral Risk Factors Surveillance System* (BRFSS) for adults, the *Pregnancy Risk Assessment Monitoring System* (PRAMS) for pregnant women and new mothers, and the *Child Health Survey* (CHS) for kids aged 1 to 14. The data available at this time cannot answer all of the important questions about whether or not marijuana use patterns are changing as a result of legalization. However, the data presented here provides a snapshot that allows us to begin to measure the public health impact....We also found moderate evidence that maternal use of marijuana during pregnancy is associated with decreased growth in exposed offspring."[5]

Highlights from the report show serious changes since 2014, when retail marijuana businesses began operating in Colorado, including traffic deaths: "A 32 percent increase in marijuana-related traffic deaths in just one year from 2013. Driving under the influence: Toxicology reports with positive marijuana results of active THC for primarily driving under the influence have increased 45 percent. Colorado youth usage (ages 12 to 17) ranks 56 percent higher than the national average. ER visits: A 29 percent increase in the number of marijuana-related emergency room visits. Hospitalizations: A 38 percent increase in the number of marijuana-related hospitalizations. Poison control: Marijuana-only related exposures increased 72 percent in only one year."[5]

Statements made by Colorado District Attorney Dan May, during a press conference in July 2017 resulted in the following headline: *Colorado official: 'Marijuana is gateway drug to homicide'*. The press conference, which included Colorado Attorney General Cynthia Coffman, announced the indictment of 13 owners, managers, and employees of "Hoppz' Crops", a marijuana head shop in Colorado Springs. According to Coffman, the store sold cigarette lighters and other cheap merchandise at a high price while offering grams of marijuana for free. This scam covered up over a half million in retail sales of marijuana.

At the press conference, District Attorney Dan May said marijuana is the "gateway drug to homicide."—"Colorado Springs Police Department put out this year we had 22 homicides in Colorado Springs last year, 2016. Eight of those were directly marijuana. That isn't somebody just using marijuana, that is somebody being murdered over legal marijuana grow in their house. Murdered over an illegal marijuana grow."

May went on to say local authorities are overwhelmed with trying to stop the crime involved with marijuana.

"Marijuana is pouring out of Colorado," May said. "It's much more valuable in the streets of New York City than it is in the streets of Denver. Colorado's system is terrible."[6,7]

11. Potency

Canada's largest publicly traded marijuana company, Canopy Growth, told a *CTV News* reporter in February of 2017, that approximately one third of the company's customers were asking for moderate to high levels of THC products.[1] In response to consumer demand the company reported that it was working on a medi-pot with 27% THC and mentioned that the company had submitted the product to the Canadian government for regulatory approval.[1]

"Our kids are getting access to the potent marijuana edibles. Adults are absolutely shocked," reported Diane Clarson of Smart Colorado.[2] Of the four states that had legalized marijuana for non-medical use as of 2014, none of the ballot initiatives that were placed before American voters included distinctions on the level of THC that would be accepted for products released to the market under legalization.

THC levels in marijuana averaged about 4% 30 years ago, and has now risen to 17.1%.[3] In recent years, THC levels exceed 20% in many of the retail edibles, and can reach 95% in the case of concentrates.[3] Hashish oil, a solvent-extracted liquid, is consumed by smoking, vaporization, or used as a food additive. Consumers report and scientific study substantiates, an increase in addictive behaviours and withdrawal symptoms are associated with high THC levels in hashish oil.[4, 5]

"As the drug becomes stronger, we are seeing clear connections between marijuana use and depression, psychotic behavior, schizophrenia, bipolar disorder and anxiety disorder."[6] —Dr. Eric Voth, Chairman of the Institute on Global Drug Policy.

In 2016, the emergency room at Providence St. Peter Hospital in Olympia Washington attended on average two cases of marijuana-induced psychosis cases every day from the use of high potency marijuana from dabbing.[7] Dabbing involves smoking a form of concentrated marijuana with a high percentage of THC. The negative outcomes can include extreme paranoia, reports of hallucinations, and or delusionary thoughts including suicidal ideation.[7]

A young man mistakenly ate a marijuana bar, intended as six servings. The 4:20 bar label read "Milk Chocolate 65 Milligrams of THC", across the front of the packaging, with an image of a tree and the words "evergreen herbal". The product was made by the Venice Cookie Company. The young man's mother wrote in an article for *Motherlode*, posted on *NYTimes.com*, that her son was cooking dinner and eating a chocolate bar when he suddenly did not feel well. He called 911, thinking he was dying. He also called his parents. His mother recalled that at the time of the incident her son could not remember the names of his siblings.[8]

In 2014, a 19 year old youth began by eating a single piece of a THC cookie, as directed by the sales clerk who had sold him the product.[9] He preceded within the next hour, not having feeling any effects from the first portion, to consume the rest of the cookie. During the next 2 hours, he reportedly exhibited erratic speech and hostile behaviors.[9] Approximately 3.5 hours after the initial portion, and 2.5 hours after consuming the remainder of the cookie, he jumped off a fourth floor balcony and died from trauma.[9] The autopsy found marijuana intoxication as a chief contributing factor.[10] The young man, it was reported, had never used marijuana before, and had no history of alcohol abuse, illicit drug use, or mental illness.[9] The autopsy report revealed that there were no other drugs in his system at the time of his death.[10]

In 2015, a 23 year old man's family linked his suicide death to marijuana edible products. The young man and his cousin, reportedly purchased $78.00 worth of peach tart marijuana candies, each containing 10mg of THC.[11] After eating at least five of the candies, the 23 year old began to talk incoherently. That evening he shot himself dead.[11]

In October of 2014, the Colorado Department of Public Health and Environment recommended a ban on retail marijuana edibles, after reported incidents of harm. The Colorado government has limited the amount of THC in edible products to 10mg per serving with a maximum of 10 servings per package.

The Colorado Department of Revenue reported that there were over three hundred varieties of candy-flavored marijuana available for sale in the state. The report was issued in February of 2015 and included the following additional information: "109,578 pounds of medical marijuana flowers were sold for the year to date along with 38,660 pounds of retail marijuana flowers; 1,964,917 units of medical marijuana edibles were sold and 2,850,733 units of retail edibles products. In total, there was approximately 5.59 million units of edible and non-edible medical marijuana infused products and retail marijuana products sold in 2014. There were 833 retail establishments with licenses and 1,416 medical business licenses as of December 2014.[12]

In May 2014, the Marijuana Enforcement implemented required potency tests for retail marijuana products sold in Colorado to ensure retail marijuana products complied with the new limits. In 2014, pursuant to the medical marijuana code, there were no requirements for medical marijuana businesses to test any medical marijuana products produced at licensed premises.[13]

ACCESS TO MARIJUANA   Thirty eight percent of Colorado youth report they got their marijuana products from a friend who obtained it legally: 23% reported from their parents, 22% from the black market, 9% from medical marijuana dispensaries, 4% from medical marijuana cardholders, and 3% from retail marijuana stores (2015).[14] It is estimated that one third of high school seniors in Colorado got their marijuana supply from a third party's prescription.[15]

ADDICTED Thirty percent of marijuana users in America meet the criteria for marijuana use disorders, according to data released in October of 2015, from the National Institute on Alcohol and Alcoholism (NIAAA).[16]

In 2013, the American Psychiatric Association added cannabis withdrawal to the fifth edition of the *Diagnostic and Statistical Manual of Mental Disorders* (DSM), as a recognized condition. Cannabis-use disorders are defined in *The Diagnostic and Statistical Manual of Mental Disorders* (DSM-5; APA, 2013) and in the *International Statistical Classification of Diseases and*

Related Health Problems (ICD-10; WHO, 1992). The classifications also describe a specific cannabis withdrawal syndrome, which can occur within 24 hours of consumption.[17]

For cannabis withdrawal syndrome to be diagnosed, the person must report at least two mental symptoms (e.g. irritability, restlessness, anxiety, depression, aggressiveness, loss of appetite, sleep disturbances) and at least one physical symptom (e.g. pain, shivering, sweating, elevated body temperature, chills). These symptoms are most intense in the first week of abstinence but can persist for as long as a month.[18]

"Those treated for addiction to cannabis (marijuana) had a higher mortality rate (3.85) times higher than controls, higher if compared to death rate risk of cocaine use disorder (2.96), alcohol use disorder (3.83), but lower than opioid use disorder (5.71) or methamphetamine use disorder (4.67). The study demonstrates that individuals with cannabis (marijuana) use disorders have a higher mortality risk than those with diagnoses related to cocaine or alcohol, but lower mortality risk than persons with methamphetamine or opioid–related disorders."[19]
—All-cause mortality among individuals with disorders related to the use of methamphetamine: A comparative cohort study. (*Drug Alcohol Depend.* October 2012)

AllTranz Inc., a pharmaceutical company, announced on November 3, 2009 that it has been awarded a $4 million research grant from the National Institute on Drug Abuse to advance the company's transdermal tetrahydrocannabinol (THC) patch for the treatment of marijuana dependence and withdrawal.[20]

THE DEVELOPING BRAIN ON MARIJUANA   Data gathered from Northwestern Medical Center, Massachusetts General, and Harvard University, confirms that three-dimensional brain "changes" are found in casual weekly or biweekly marijuana users.[21] The changes were predominately in adolescent brains, but visible changes have been noted up until the age of thirty.[22]

The age of risk for the very serious mental health outcome of cannabis use, chronic psychosis, begins to taper off considerably after age 30.[23] "The risk for addiction diminishes significantly with maturity."[24] —Hall and Degenhardt, 2009

"Why the risk for addiction is greater when the brain is still developing can be understood through its effect on the reward system of the brain, which relies heavily on the release of dopamine during the performance of activities that should bring pleasure. Cannabis stimulates the release of dopamine, eventually leading to diminished dopamine release (van de Giessen et al., 2017). The effect is most easily detected in those who begin cannabis use at younger ages (Urban et al., 2012) in whom cessation of cannabis use would be expected to elicit stronger cravings in those whose neurodevelopment was completed in the presence of THC than in those whose neurodevelopment occurred in the absence of THC."[25] —Christine L. Miller, Ph.D.

CONSULT TO THE GOVERNMENT OF CANADA "Research suggests that cannabis use during adolescence may be associated with effects on the development of the brain. Use before a certain age comes with increased risk. Yet current science is not definitive on a safe age for cannabis use, so science alone cannot be relied upon to determine the age of lawful purchase. Recognizing that persons under the age of 25 represent the segment of the population most likely to consume cannabis and to be charged with a cannabis possession offence, and in view of the Government's intention to move away from a system that criminalizes the use of cannabis, it is important in setting a minimum age that we do not disadvantage this population. There was broad agreement among participants and the Task Force that setting the bar for legal access too high could result in a range of unintended consequences, such as leading those consumers to continue to purchase cannabis on the illicit market.

For these reasons, the Task Force is of the view that the federal government should set a minimum age of 18 for the legal sale of cannabis, leaving it to provinces and territories to set a higher minimum age should they wish to do so. To mitigate harms between the ages of 18 and 25, a period of continued brain development, governments should do all that they can to discourage and delay cannabis use. Robust preventive measures, including advertising restrictions and public education, all of which are addressed later in this chapter, are seen as key to discouraging use by this age group."[26] —Canadian Task Force (2016)

"The principal difference between legality and illegality is the number of victims, which will be far greater if the drug is legalised."[27] —Peter Hitchens (UK)

"One adverse outcome of cannabis use that may not be directly tempered by setting the age limit at 30 is the increased risk for suicide (increased about 5 to 7-fold in cannabis users; Arendt et al., 2013; Silins et al., 2014; Kvitland et al., 2015; even after a prior history of depression is corrected for—Clarke et al., 2014), because the age of risk for suicide does not peak until middle age. However, there would be an indirect benefit because the risk of addiction would be diminished by setting the lawful age at 30, thereby limiting the number of heavy users in the age group at most risk."[28] —Christine L. Miller, Ph.D.

The Canadian *Cannabis Act Bill C-45* reads: "The term 'young person' is defined to mean: for the purpose of sections 8, 9, and 12, an individual who is 12 years of age or older but under 18 years of age; and for the purposes of any other provisions in this Act, an individual who is under 18 years of age."[29]

"Part 1, Section 1, Division 1 Criminal Activities, reads at 8 (1)Possession : Unless authorized under this Act, it is prohibited; for an individual who is 18 years of age or older to possess, in a public place, cannabis of one or more classes of cannabis the total amount of which, as determined in accordance with Schedule 3, is equivalent to more than 30g of dried cannabis; for an individual who is 18 years of age or older to possess any cannabis that they know is illicit cannabis; for a young person to possess cannabis of one or more classes of cannabis the total amount of which, as determined in accordance with Schedule 3, is equivalent to more than 5g of dried cannabis."[29]

What course of action is called for when a Canadian at the age of 12 is found in possession of more than 5g of marijuana (roughly $50.00), will have to be determined. *Bill C-45* would see many of the restrictions under the existing *Controlled Drugs and Substances Act* remain in effect regarding the selling, producing, importing and exporting of marijuana outside the proposed regulated guidelines. For persons caught distributing or selling marijuana to minors, *Bill C-45* includes a penalty for this offense that amounts to a maximum of 14 years' imprisonment. As the bulk of the current marijuana market is youth, the Canadian family and educational institutions are facing challenging times ahead; as 18 year olds are granted legal access to 30g of marijuana and will in all probability use with friends, and younger siblings. They will also be the targets for drug traffickers, as will their younger counterparts.

MARIJUANA AND POST TRAUMATIC STRESS DISORDER The USA Veterans Affairs Administration recognizes that individuals with PTSD, who smoke marijuana, make significantly less progress in overcoming their condition than those that don't use.[30]

PTSD patients are already more vulnerable to psychosis and clinicians have witnessed psychotic breaks in PTSD patients who begin using marijuana products.[31] "While the symptoms that afflict PTSD patients (anxiety, depression, panic) may be temporarily relieved while the subjects are 'high', these very same symptoms are exacerbated in the long run."[32] —Christine L. Miller, Ph.D.

A study published by the *Journal of Psychiatric Research*, *Cannabis use disorder and suicide attempts in Iraq/Afghanistan-era veterans*, found that marijuana-dependent Iraq/Afghanistan-era veterans had an increased risk of suicidal thoughts and attempted suicide. More than 3,000 veterans were sampled. The study design controlled for extraneous factors including PTSD, depression, alcohol dependence, and other drug disorders.[33]

A 2017 report, from the National Academies of Sciences (NAS), found only limited evidence that marijuana or cannabinoids could be effective in treating symptoms of PTSD.[34] The NAS report also showed a strong association between marijuana use and society anxiety disorders, depressive disorders, and schizophrenia.[34]

A study in 2015 from researchers at Yale University also showed a connection between marijuana use and PTSD symptoms and violent behaviour.[35] Dr. Samuel Wilkinson, an author of the study, told the *New Haven Register* (Connecticut) that he queried why states have approved marijuana for PTSD and a variety of other conditions, without controlled studies and approval by the U.S. FDA.[36] The study reads: "The results of our study provide no support for the hypothesis that marijuana is associated with general improvement in PTSD symptoms, and the observed associations suggest that it may actually worsen PTSD symptoms or nullify the benefits of specialized, intensive treatment. Especially in light of the adverse health effects of marijuana use, data indicate that providers should be cautious or even avoidant in using this agent to treat PTSD."[37]

The U.S. Department of Veterans Affairs recently reported that approximately 20 veterans die by suicide each day in the United States.[38] "It is distressing to realize that many veterans suffering from PTSD have been sold the false promise that marijuana use can ease their symptoms, when in fact the science shows it's just the opposite," said SAM President Kevin A. Sabet, Ph.D.[39]

Since 2008, Veterans Affairs Canada (VAC) has provided coverage for the cost of marijuana for medical purposes to veterans, who obtained the product in accordance with Health Canada regulations. "Marijuana has harmful effects and there's no proof it helps with post-traumatic stress disorder," said (former) Canadian Veterans Affairs Minister Erin O'Toole in an interview with the *CBC* on May 13, 2015.[40]

According to Veterans Affair Canada, the federal department spent $5.2 million on medical marijuana for veterans in the fiscal year of 2014 with almost 3.4 million, or 65% going to veterans in Atlantic Canada.[41]

On April 1, 2014, Health Canada released new regulations allowing private producers, licensed by Health Canada, to supply Canadians with marijuana who have authorization from a physician. The licensed producers were left to determine the price to charge the recipients.

Commercial suppliers had been charging up to $14 per gram, almost triple the federal government's estimate.[42] The government report also revealed that just one doctor had written 29% of the prescriptions for marijuana for medical purposes accessed by the veterans for 2014-2015. The Federal Government paid $44.5 million to cover marijuana for medical purposes to veterans in 2015-2016, which was an increase of three times the amount paid out for combined amounts for the two previous years.

The Minister of Veteran Affairs for Canada announced a crack-down on not only the amount dispensed but also the price per gram the government would pay as the program moved forward.[43,44]

Canadians who meet clinical criteria for PTSD, due to trauma experienced during military service, as a first responder or police, or as the result of violence and/or sexual assault are to take part in a study that is scheduled to conclude in spring 2018. The study is sponsored by Tilray.[45]

Victims of trauma, will often use mind-altering drugs, including marijuana and alcohol to disassociate, or attempt to escape overwhelming feelings of tension or fear. Dr. Janina Fisher, Ph.D., writes of marijuana and heroin as having the power to create a numbing effect. Her paper, *Traumatic Abuse and Addiction* explains the dynamic of compensatory strategies aimed at self-regulation from the experience of trauma in detail.[46] When marijuana or heroin are used and the result is too much disassociation, other drugs may then be used as a counter measure, including cocaine or opiates. Some trauma victims, as do other members of the public including the young, self-regulate with marijuana products and will go on to experience anxiety instead of the desired numbing or go on to become addicted.

The scientific literature provides a very strong case for abstinence based treatment for patients with PTSD.[47] If addiction recovery strengthens trauma recovery it is questioned what, if any role marijuana products can ever play in the reducing the crippling anguish of trauma.

12. Rates of Use

"The original epidemic of illicit drug use in the 1960s began on the nation's college campuses and the spread downward in age. By way of contrast, Monitoring the Future has shown that the relapse phase in the 1990s first manifested itself among secondary school students and then started moving upward in age as those cohorts matured."[1] —MTF

From the early 1990s until 1997, marijuana use rose sharply among secondary school students, as did their use of other illicit drugs, though at a more gradually pace.[1] Monitoring the Future 1992 survey results for eighth and twelfth graders showed the perception of risk in using drugs beginning to decline, as did the proportion of students saying they disapproved of use.[1] "As we suggested then, those reversals indeed presaged an end to the improvements in the drug situation that the nation may be taking for granted."[1] —MTF

"There are several possible and interconnected explanations for the turnaround and decline in perceived risk of marijuana use during the early 1990s. First, some of the forces that gave rise to the earlier increases in perceived risk became less influential: Because of lower use levels overall, fewer students had opportunities for vicarious learning by observing firsthand the effects of heavy marijuana use among their peers; Media coverage of the harmful effects of drug use, as well as of incidents resulting from drug use (particularly marijuana), decreased substantially in the early 1990s (as has been documented by media surveys of national news programs); Media coverage of the antidrug advertising campaign of the *Partnership for a Drug-Free America* also declined appreciably (as documented by both the *Partnership* and our own data from 12th graders on their levels of recalled exposure to such ads); Congressional funding for drug abuse prevention programs and curricula in the schools was cut appreciably in the early 1990s; and the first Gulf War in 1990-1991 diverted attention from domestic concerns, including drug use, among policy makers and the media.

In addition, forces encouraging use became more visible; in particular, a number of rap, grunge, and rock groups started to sing the praises of using marijuana (and sometimes other drugs), perhaps influencing young people to think that using drugs might not be so dangerous after all. Finally, the drug experiences of many parents may have inhibited them from discussing drugs with their children, and may have caused them uncertainty in knowing how to handle the apparent hypocrisy of telling their children not to do what they themselves had done as teens. We believe that all of these factors may have contributed to the resurgence of marijuana use in the 1990s."[1] —MTF

PARENTAL ATTITUDES According to a 2010 national survey by SAMHSA, youth aged 12 to 17, were less likely to use a substance if they believed their parents would strongly disapprove and this was particularly true for tobacco and marijuana.[2]

The National Center on Addiction and Substance Abuse (CASA) at Columbia University, issued a National Study in June 29, 2011: "5% (10 million) of all high school students in America have used addictive substances including tobacco, alcohol, marijuana or cocaine; 1 in 5 of them meets the medical criteria for addiction. Forty-six percent of children under the age of 18 (34.4 million) live in a household where someone 18 or older is smoking, drinking excessively, misusing prescription drugs or using illegal drugs. Less than half (42.6%) of parents list refraining from smoking cigarettes, drinking alcohol, using marijuana, misusing prescription drugs or using other illicit drugs as one of their top three concerns for their teens; almost 21% say that marijuana is a harmless drug."[3]

December 2016 federal data shows, Colorado leading the nation in terms of the percentage of teens using marijuana.[4] The U.S. Substance Abuse and Mental Health Services Administration reports that in 2014-15 more than 11% of Coloradans aged 12-17 had used marijuana in the past month. Colorado survey results show 48% of Colorado high school students saw marijuana as risky in 2015, down from 54% two years earlier.[5]

THE PRICE OF MARIJUANA A report commissioned by the State of California pre-election 2010, concluded that legalization could usher in lower prices for marijuana, as much as 80% lower, and that such a drop in prices could well increase consumption and demand.[6] The Rand Corporation, testifying before the State of California in 2010, cautioned that tax revenues could not be adequately calculated and were subject to the influence of the rate of tax evasion and the activities of the black market, along with other factors.[6] In Colorado, the average wholesale price has fallen since legal sales to adults started in January 2014.[7]

SOCIAL FACTORS AND INITIATION "In developed countries the major social and contextual factors that increase the likelihood of initiation of cannabis use are; drug availability, the use of tobacco and alcohol at an early age, and social norms that are tolerant of alcohol and drug use. Overall, people from socially disadvantaged backgrounds are more likely to use illicit drugs, although illicit drugs can also be commonly used in specific subgroups and party settings.

Family factors that are found to increase the risk of illicit drug use during adolescence include the poor quality of parent-child interaction and parent-child relationships, parental conflict, and parental and sibling drug use. However, there is no absolute relationship and not all adolescents growing up in families with these risk factors become illicit drug users. Individual risk factors that increase the risk include: male gender, the personality traits of novelty and sensation seeking, peer early oppositional behaviour and conduct disorders in childhood, poor school performance, low commitment to education and early school leaving, inadequate sleep.

Other factors influencing use include: Associating with anti-social and drug-using peers is a strong predictor of adolescent alcohol and drug use. In developed countries protective factors in childhood and adolescence are found to be positive family environments. Young adults who experienced strong parental support during adolescence are less likely to develop drug-use problems.

Perceptions of parental care play a key role in predicting

cannabis use. Good family management—encompassing effective monitoring, discipline, reward systems, reinforcement, etc.—is associated with lower rates of substance use among young adults."[8] —UNODC (2015)

"The youngster who is quietly stoned during school does not learn math or grammar or biology, or how to cope with boredom, pressure and discipline. He will not have much going for him when he leaves the protective nest—home and high school—as an 18 year old. The real world out there is tough and it does not make excuses for the supposed young adult who befuddled his adolescence with marijuana or any other drugs, for the youngster who messed up or opted out of his apprenticeship to adulthood. Trust your gut instincts as parents: you have every right to worry about the use of any psychoactive drugs, especially illegal drugs, by your child."[9] —Marsha Schuchard, *The Family versus the Drug Culture*, First PRIDE Conference, Atlanta, Georgia, (1978)

HOCKEY AND DRUGS DO NOT MIX Concerned parents have approached hockey association leadership seeking guidance on how best to respond to the increased use of marijuana by young players both on and off the ice. "Drugs and hockey do not mix," responded Stephen Heisler of JuniorHockey.com.

Former North American Hockey League bench boss Chuck Linkenheld weighed in on the issue of drug use in junior hockey: "Certainly we can't ignore youth hockey and particularly high school age players. In my opinion this is where it starts. If you do any kind of drugs at this age get out of sports and go hang out with someone else until it is time for rehab! Parents need to pull their head out of the sand and do a little investigating and spying. Don't make it so damn easy for your potential junior and college player to ruin their hockey career and maybe their life.

If you know they smoke, then suspend them yourself. Listen I didn't grow up blind and stupid and I know kids make mistakes like we all did but parents can keep them from making the same mistake twice and creating public embarrassment and headline news. Do the math. If I catch my kid and I spend $10,000 per year on hockey I can save all that cash for their eventual rehab."[10]

The tough part of being a parent is sometimes you have to be the "cop", you have to be the one to draw the line on drugs. Hockey or no hockey is a choice that may have to be made.

OFFERING A WAY OUT "I taught biology for over 30 years in one of the pilot schools and was responsible for drug education. I saw that the boys were greatly taken by the very friendly dogs (spaniels) especially when, in a demonstration, they correctly identified the member of staff (a very popular young man) as having had drugs placed on his person. Not only did this scheme act as a deterrent but in my many years of contact with boys (11 to 18) I learned that the vast majority (over 95%) did not want ever to take drugs. What they wanted and asked from me were reliable and complete scientific facts about drugs and their potentially dangerous effects on their brains and bodies so that they were armed with an excuse to refuse. The welcome random dog visits gave them another reason to say 'No'."

Children deserve to experience a safe and creative education in a secure learning environment in order to reach their full potential. Recently, one obstacle has been the presence of illegal drugs in schools and the targeting of school children by dealers, sometimes their own peer group. An initiative to introduce drug dogs by our school police liaison officer in Buckinghamshire (UK) resulted in a pilot scheme in which 6 very different schools took part. Lengthy deliberation by head teachers, the local education authority, police and others took place.

The approach was supportive rather than punitive but not a soft option. Clear disciplinary measures were in place in the schools with referral for counselling and rehabilitation and all visits were carried out in the presence of police officers. Robust drug education programmes were also in place. Parents were advised and letters sent home. They were given the opportunity to ask questions, to object and request that their child be excused from taking part. Staff members were generally informed at staff meetings. Pupils were informed in classes and at assemblies.

The pilot scheme was fully put into operation in the 2003-04 academic year. Of those who thought it was a good idea, 98% of parents, 92% of staff and 82% of pupils agreed. Almost the same numbers thought it should continue and 82% of pupils, 94% of parents and 81% of staff thought there should be no prior warning of the visits. All parties generally rated the drugs dog initiative to have been very successful and great emphasis was placed on the merits of continuing the scheme."[11] —Mary Brett

A study set out in 2015 to search *YouTube* for videos about edible marijuana products and review the access to the videos by youth.[12] Fifty-one identified videos had been seen by greater than 9 million viewers, with only 7 having a restriction to viewers 18 years of age and older. The researchers concluded that edible marijuana videos were easy to find, and the videos often instructed on how to cook, and the material was presented in an entertaining way that could make the activity appealing to viewers.[12]

"We can survive if we eat candy for an entire day, but if we put the greenmarkets out of business along the way, all that's left is candy. Give your kid a tablet, a game, and some chicken fingers for dinner. It's easier than talking to him. Read the short articles, the ones with pictures, it's simpler than digging deep."
—Seth Godin

13. Hollyweed

On New Year's Day 2017, Californians woke up to find that their iconic hillside sign "Hollywood" had been the target of a publicity pot stunt. The sign now read "Hollyweed".

The electorate over the past twenty years has been ever-more drawn into the contested issue of marijuana policy. They have been asked to vote on marijuana ballot initiatives and to vote for individuals running for public office, who if elected, could bring major changes to long-standing drug policies that continue to be supported the world over.

An estimated eighty-five million people were eligible to vote on a marijuana ballot initiative in the US presidential election of 2016, an election that saw Californians vote to permit adults legal access to marijuana, with some restrictions, and they were prompted to do so by big money interests.

"Ballot initiatives originated in the 1900s in California to give citizens power over corporate influence on the legislature. But collecting signatures to place an initiative on the ballot has become such a big business that only big businesses—or billionaires—can afford to participate. Gone are the days when an idealistic group of volunteers went door-to-door collecting signatures from neighbors and friends to support a ballot

d killing other innocent drivers on the road. *AUMA*
hose 21 and older to grow up to six indoor plants.
ll anyone know if someone is growing six or sixteen
de their home? More importantly, if the person
rowing is a juvenile, the punishment is an infrac-
, juveniles face only an infraction for possession,
 for selling or for transporting ANY amount of
hus, the *AUMA* actually encourages the entry of
 the industry. These issues are only some of the
 arise from the legalization of marijuana and the
e *AUMA*. These concerns must be considered
lligent decision is made on whether to support or
easure."[3]

Initiative specified that the manufacturing butane
 be a felony which carried a penalty of a $50,000
 to seven year jail sentence.[4]

o the California Drug Endangered Children
dvocacy Center (DEC-TAC), there have been
 forty one THC extraction laboratories recorded
 of April 6, 2015.[5] DEC-TAC reports children
eventy-two THC extraction laboratories, result-
 injured, and the death of 3 children.[5] Further,
ts 140 adults were injured, and 41 adults were
 extraction laboratory explosions.[5]

26, 2016, on the *CBS* show *60 Minutes*,
 Colorado, John Hickenlooper offered his
states: "My recommendation has been that
owly and probably wait a couple of years,"
 sure that we get some good vertical studies
 there isn't a dramatic increase in teenage

measure. Today, whole businesses exist to collect signatures at so much per name, and they usually collect double those required to guarantee enough will be valid. In California, 365,880 valid signatures were required to place a measure on the November 2016 ballot at a cost of $2.72-$11.31 per signature. Few initiatives pass without significant advertising budgets to persuade citizens to vote yes, so only the rich can afford to sponsor a successful ballot initiative. And few ordinary citizens can raise enough money to oppose it. Nowhere can this be seen more clearly than with the three billionaires who financed the marijuana legalization movement."[1]
—National Families in Action, *Tracking the Money* (2017)

Funding in support of the 2016 California ballot initiative, *Proposition 64*, came substantially from several billionaires.[2] Total spent by the proponents was $35,667,001.00; the amount spent by the opponents was $2,512,438.00.[2]

"Proponents' contributions included: 3 billionaires giving $22,829,841.00; from within the state monies received from individuals $174,158.00; individuals within the marijuana industry $2,000,000.00; non-individuals $90,646.00; non-individuals in the marijuana industry $9,206,499.00; out-of-state money from individuals $29,485.00; out-of-state individuals in the marijuana industry $1,250,000.00; out-of-state non-individuals $25,757.00 and out-of-state non-individuals in the marijuana industry $60,015.00.; with out-of-country contributions amounting to $600.00.

In 1996, the ballot initiative *Proposition 215*, seeking legal access to medi-pot in the state of California, the Drug Policy Alliance raised $2,479,680 to opponents $33,612.00.

Shortly after *Proposition 215* passed, a representative of

Zimmerman and Markham, a professional campaign firm, spoke at NORML's annual conference to explain how the campaign was won: *We came in with outside money. We bought the signatures. We had television advertising. We had sophisticated press strategies.*"[1]
—National Families in Action, *Tracking the Money* (2017)

A letter written by Bonnie M. Dumanis, Attorney General of San Diego County, before the decision by the electorate on the proposal to legalize marijuana for non-medical uses in California raises key aspects of the plan: "On November 2, 2015, proponents for the legalization of marijuana, including Sean Parker, submitted a proposed state-wide ballot initiative with a request for title and summary. The proposed initiative was assigned number 15-0103, and was titled, *The Control, Regulate,* and *Tax Adult Use of Marijuana Act.* It is also known as the *Parker Initiative,* and the *Adult Use of Marijuana Act* or the *(AUMA).* An amended version of the proposed initiative was submitted on December 7, 2015. Title and Summary were prepared on January 6, 2016. If passed by the voters, the initiative would legalize the possession of one ounce of marijuana and the cultivation of six plants by adults, 21 years of age and over. The Office of the San Diego County District Attorney has not taken a position on the initiative. However, there are concerns that are worth noting."[3]

The Dumanis letter continues: "Proponents of the initiative claim that 'by bringing marijuana into a regulated and legitimate market, *AUMA* creates a transparent and accountable system. This will help police crackdown on the underground black market that currently benefits violent drug cartels and transnational gangs, which are making billions from marijuana trafficking and jeopardizing public safety.' However, it is

a mistake to infer that cartels a
get out of the drug dealing busi
geoning multi-billion dollar a y

Cartels and gangs don't pl
don't obey regulations and la
their innovative smuggling st
our public land to grow thou
plants. 'The competitive ad
stems from their proficiency
gling, none of which are es
said Ethan Nadelmann, di

While the trafficking
amine is the main focus
juana that has long prov
drug cartels. More tha
billion out of $13.8 bi
juana sales, according
Drug Control Policy.

There are no ind
cocaine to become
greater criminal pre
rise in California a
legalized marijuana

AUMA allocate
and adopt DUID
protocols. Currer
is no clarificatior
the person is a
and evidence ba
meantime, peo

injuring a
will allow
How w
plants insi
doing the g
tion. In fac
for growing
marijuana.
juveniles int
concerns tha
passage of th
before an inte
oppose this m
The Parker
hash oil would
fine and a thre
According
Training and A
four hundred an
in California as
were present at s
ing in 12 childrer
DEC-TAC repor
killed due to THC
On October
the Governor of
opinion to other
they should go sl
—"And let's make
to make sure that

usage, that there isn't a significant increase in abuse like while driving. We don't see it yet, but the data is not perfect. And we don't have enough data yet to make that decision."[6]

"A dangerous precedent is set by approval processes that are effectively achieved through the popular vote of citizens who are not expert judges of medical efficacy, abuse potential, or ethics of the doctor-patient relationship. Popular vote is also risky because the public is then at the mercy of pressures from groups who are using medical marijuana as a beachhead for generalised legal access to marijuana."[7] —Gregory Pike, Adelaide Centre for Bioethics and Culture, Australia

14. Regulate and Tax

THE TAX CARD "We cannot afford to forget the painful lessons of our national experience with Big Tobacco, which for decades lied to Americans about its products and marketed an addictive, harmful drug to minority communities and young people to make money. No amount of tax revenue will ever undo the heavy price our society paid for that mistake," stated Rafael Lemaitre, former Associate Director for Public Affairs for the White House Drug Policy Office, during the Obama administration.[1]

Alcohol costs: "According to *The Economic Costs of Alcohol Abuse Report*, alcoholism costs U.S. employers 500 million lost work days per year (NIDA 2000). The cost of alcohol abuse in the United Sates is at least $185 billion annually. In other words, for every dollar we bring in, we spend ten. Why are we holding this up as a revenue model?"[2] —Jo McGuire, Colorado

One in ten people die an alcohol related death—between the ages of 20-64.[3]

"Canadians are asking for it, Canadians believe it's time to have marijuana legalized," (Angus) McNeil (MP Government of Canada) commented. To which he added: "I'm sure there will be tax revenue, yes."[4] —Global News 2016

"If they're looking at pot as something that might swoop in and save them they need to keep looking," said Joseph Henchman, an analyst who studied marijuana tax collection for the Tax Foundation, a nonpartisan tax think tank.[5]

"Because the data required for formal cost-benefit analysis is not available at this time, invoking fiscal rhetoric to advance the legalization agenda is not merely irresponsible, it is also deceitful. In effect, it defies transparency, misdirects public debate, and belies a corporate purpose to privatize profits and socialize losses, subordinating the interests of the taxpayers to those of the marijuana industry."[5] —David G. Evans, Esq., Executive Director, Drug Free Projects Coalition

In 2016, the State of Arizona made $30 million in tax revenues off the $280 million generated from the sale of medi-pot.[6] Who should be paying all the related societal costs associated with the recent proliferation of marijuana in the state? Should it be the non-indulging taxpayer, the industry or the marijuana consumer? In 2016, 29 tons of marijuana for medical purposes was consumed in Arizona, more than double the amount from the previous year. 114,000 people were legally using medi-pot in Arizona as of 2016.[6]

"In a biennial report presented this week to the Santa Cruz County Board of Supervisors, country health officials found that most local emergency room visits are due to drug and alcohol abuse. The report also noted that homeless people in the county suffer from disproportionately high rates of substance abuse, which exacerbates the problem of chronic homelessness."[7] —Santa Cruz Sentinel

19.5% of California's budget is consumed by substance abuse. The annual cost to California for the 24.2% school dropouts is $46.4 billion, $392,000 per dropout. Preventing marijuana and drug use would save the state billions of dollars.[8]

THE RACIST CARD Those pushing the pro-marijuana agenda have a vested interest in keeping the conversation well away from the world of evidence based science and off the topic of health. Entangling the issue of access to pot with other "conversations of the day" is a calculated move, as is involving it in partisan politics. Many who are well positioned to speak up and out against moving public health policy in a more permissive direction have been "spooked" off the issue out of fear of appearing "political". This has in essence silenced many important voices, including many in the medical profession and public health sector.

"I went to Ferguson in a quest to be in solidarity and stand with the young organizers and affirm their leadership," said Kassandra Frederique, policy manager of the Drug Policy Alliance.[9] "We recognized this movement is similar to the work we're doing in the DPA," said Frederique. Frederique continued; "The war on drugs has always been to operationalize, institutionalize and criminalize people of color. Protecting personal sovereignty is a cornerstone of the work we do and what this movement is all about."[9]

"The 2015 US census shows that people of various race and ethnicity attend Colorado hospital emergency rooms for marijuana harms at disproportionate rates. In Colorado, in 2015 4.5% of the population were Black, and 87.5% were White. Hospital emergency room visits reflect the disproportion use of marijuana products across race and ethnic lines; White 895 attendees, Black 904, Hispanic 562, other 793, unknown 1743 based on per 100,000."[10] —Colorado Hospital Association. (2014 thru September 2015)

Battling Menthol Restrictions, R.J. Reynolds Reaches Out To Sharpton, Other Black Leaders, written by Myron Levin and published in *FairWarning*, examines how civil rights activists were drawn into the issue of proposed restrictions on menthol cigarettes.[11] If menthol cigarettes were banned, a favorite product within the black community, the argument was put forward that the result could be increased police harassment of blacks, who after the imposing of restrictions would turn to the underground market for menthol cigarettes.

"In the recent months, the company (R.J. Reynolds) has quietly enlisted black groups and leaders, including civil rights activist Rev. Al Sharpton and ex-Florida Congressman Kendrick B. Meek, to hold meetings at prominent black churches on the theme of "Decriminalizing the Black Community."—Levin reports. Speakers at the Reynolds-sponsored meetings have included John I. Dixon III, former president of the National Organization of Black Law Enforcement Executives, Neill Franklin, a former Maryland State Police narcotics officer and executive director of the Law Enforcement Action Partnership, and Art Way Colorado state director of the Drug Police Alliance reported Levine.[11]

Afro magazine published a commentary by William Jones, a master's student of public policy at George Washington University, who also led the campaign that opposed marijuana legalization in Washington D.C: "Racial disparities in arrest rates for drugs are a well-documented (and lived) reality. For decades, drug policy has contributed to skyrocketing incarceration rates among minority populations. That marijuana legalization is promoted as a victory for racial justice is ironic at best. Just look at marijuana's counterparts, the alcohol and tobacco industries. It is an unjustified reality in Black communities that a child cannot take a walk without passing a liquor store on every corner. Liquor stores in poorer, non-White neighborhoods far outnumber those in richer, White counterparts. Pot is no different, he says. Denver black and brown neighborhoods are already experiencing this. In one minority community, there is one marijuana business for every 47 residents."[12]

"We are selling freedom, not marijuana."- Richard Cowan, NORML, *USA Today* (1994). Playing the freedom card to advance marijuana legalization is right out of the pages of tobacco strategy.

In 1968 the *Virginia Slims* cigarette line was launched as a strategy to attract a broader female market. The industry's target was young women, aged 18-35, who were fashion conscious, desirous of being thin, and predominately liberal-minded. The promotional campaigns for *Virginia Slims* fit right in with the theme of women's emancipation. *Virginia Slims* are still on the market but the derogatory slogans of the last century have been retired: *You've come a long way, Baby, to get where you've got to today. You've got your own cigarette now, Baby.*[13]

In a letter dated May 18, 1979, written by a representative of the Liggett Group Inc., to the US Secretary of Health, Education and Welfare in Washington DC the issue of "free will" is raised: "With regard to your request that the cigarette industry donate ten percent of its advertising and promotion budget aimed at a campaign to inform children "that smoking is not a habit to be embraced by children", I personally believe that the mothers and fathers of this nation, whether smokers or non-smokers, should continue to have freedom of choice in the education and training of their children and have done an excellent job of their own free will....The words 'free will' have always meant a great deal to me, and in view of that belief I frankly consider your request as one which sets a very dangerous precedent with regard to the advertising of a legal product in our democratic and free enterprise society and economy."[14]

On May 31 2011, Central Park in New York City went smoke-free. Camel retaliated with full-page color ads in publications including *USA Today* that read: "NYC Smokers enjoy freedom without the flame. Smokers switch to Camel Snus and reclaim the world's greatest city." The upper right-hand corner features the Camel logo and the slogan *BREAK FREE*.[15] In small type to the left is the following industry-generated wording: "Share your support for tobacco freedom at Camel SNUS.COM/solutions." A full page color ad ran the banner message: *NYC SMOKERS RISE ABOVE THE BAN.*[15] Marijuana use, instead of offering "free will" is the antithesis of freedom for those that become addicted.[15]

A 25-year study of people, ages 13-38 from New Zealand, documented an 8 point IQ drop in weekly marijuana users.[17] This translates to a lifetime income category drop from the 50th percentile, down to the 29th percentile, a zone at which job opportunities are known to diminish.[17]

"What is already known is that in casual users, THC can disrupt focus, working memory, decision making and motivation for 24 hours. The fact that we can see these structural effects in the brain could indicate that the effects of THC are longer lasting than we previously thought."[16] —Dr. Jodi Gilman, instructor in psychology at Harvard Medical School.

PLAYING THE JOBS CARD "We see here an industry that we think has extreme growth potential," the Premier of New Brunswick Brian Gallant, told the *Guardian*.[18] The provincial government of New Brunswick invested $4 million in a loan to a marijuana manufacturing start up to help them to build a facility so that they can create in excess of 200 new jobs.[19] The provincial government also invested in a federally licensed marijuana producer by providing $990,000 in payroll rebates for the creation of dozens of jobs over the next three years.[19]

Spokespersons for the marijuana industry frequently promote the prospect of an influx of jobs and prosperity for smaller communities with marijuana industrialization. They boast that marijuana is good for business and the economy.[20, 21, 22]

The Colorado based marijuana industrialist, Bob DeGabrielle stated that marijuana legalization had created 1,300 jobs and more than sixty businesses in Pueblo County. "In so many ways, it's been an economic windfall for the community," DeGabrielle told *CBS News* on *60 Minutes*.[23] Members of the community of Pueblo Colorado fought in the 2016 cycle to shut down the marijuana industry in their county. The community interests were defeated.

JOBS MAKE HEADLINES *Tilray, medical marijuana company, creates 275 more jobs in Nanaimo, B.C.—Smith Falls celebrates Tweed's medical marijuana licence.—Marijuana industry to bring 100 jobs to the former Hershey's plant.—Spliffy Jobs in the Marijuana Industry.*[20,21,22,23]

Governor Jerry Brown interviewed by the *Washington Post* on the prospect of legalized marijuana: "How many people can get stoned and still have a great state?"[24]

On January 4, 1987, a Conrail freight locomotive travelling from Baltimore, Maryland, to Harrisburg, Pennsylvania collided with an Amtrak train carrying 600 passengers from Washington bound for Boston. Fourteen passengers and two employees (including the engineer) on the Amtrak train were killed.[25] The direct cause of the accident was reported as a failure of the Conrail engineer to stop at a stop signal, caused by the crew's judgement being impaired by the use of marijuana.[25]

"This accident (Conrail-Amtrak Jan.4/1987) led Congress to pass legislation authorizing mandatory random testing for all employees in 'safety sensitive' jobs in industries regulated by the D.O.T. (Department of Transportation)."[26] —Alan MacMillan, retired locomotive engineer.

Any person holding a safety sensitive job is responsible, under US law, to provide a safe work environment for their co-workers and the public, therefore the use of marijuana is not permitted and individual state marijuana initiatives have no bearing on the federal legislation for 'safety-sensitive jobs'.

"What no one (especially the soon to be legal "drug dealers") is telling you, is that if you smoke/eat/drink/inhale or in any way ingest marijuana, you can never work in the transportation industry.

You cannot drive or dispatch or work on trains; you cannot fly commercial (or military) aircraft or be an air traffic controller; you cannot be a bus, long-haul truck or taxi driver; you cannot be in command of a ship or a tour boat operator, school bus drivers, train engineers, subway operators, aircraft maintenance personnel, transit fire-armed security personnel, ship captains, and pipeline emergency response personnel, among others.

You also cannot become a doctor or a nurse; you cannot work in law enforcement or the fire department. You cannot go into the military or the Coast Guard. You cannot hold a safety sensitive job anywhere, as all of these occupations now require not only pre-employment drug screening, but both random drug testing and drug testing if you are involved in an accident or an incident involving any kind of post-incident investigation. In the transportation industry, you don't get a second chance: caught once in a random drug test, you're fired. Period. I watched a co-worker once, married, 3 children and a house mortgage—get fired for drug use, his career over."[26]
—Alan MacMillan

The Transportation Safety Board listed marijuana use as a contributing cause of a fatal plane crash in 2011.[27] Two people, the pilot age 28 and a passenger age 54, were killed in the crash, and two others were seriously injured.[27] The Transportation Safety Board said that the amount of THC discovered in the pilot's bloodstream would have impaired his ability to make decisions and his ability to perform his pilot duties.[27]

"The Department of Transportation's Drug and Alcohol Testing Regulation (*49 CFR Part 40*) does not authorize the use of Schedule I drugs, including marijuana, for any reason. Therefore, Medical Review Officers (MROs) will not verify a drug test as negative based upon learning that the employee used "recreational marijuana" when states have passed "recreational marijuana" initiatives. We also firmly reiterate that an MRO will not verify a drug test negative based upon information that a physician recommended that the employee use "medical marijuana" when states have passed "medical marijuana" initiatives. It is important to note that marijuana remains a drug listed in Schedule I of the Controlled Substances Act. It remains unacceptable for any safety-sensitive employee subject to drug testing under the Department of Transportation's drug testing regulations to use marijuana."[28] —USA Department of Transportation, (2017)

"The Department of Transportation conducts urine tests for marijuana metabolites and other drugs, that will be positive for multiple days, whereas the blood level could only show marijuana used hours before the test. What is good practise for airplane pilots, airplane mechanics, train operators, bus drivers, ship operators, could well be the best policy for all persons driving automobiles." —Alan MacMillan

15. The Penalty Box

POSSESSION One point of argument raised by pro-marijuana voices is that by marijuana remaining illegal the law incarcerates unnecessarily. Otherwise law abiding citizens, who are not breaking a legitimate law but rather using "effective" medicine and possessing "non-toxic", "non-harmful, "natural" and "pure" products, are unfairly being imposed with penalties. [1, 2, 3, 4]

"People who are already vulnerable are affected disproportionately; evidence suggests that police often use the charge of cannabis possession as an easy way of harassing or making life difficult for marginalized populations."[5] —CAMH, *Cannabis Policy Framework Canada*. If law enforcement officers are misusing the law to harass people, they can be stopped and should be. This argument is not a valid case for moving to more permissive drug policies.

US Federal data from the Bureau of Justice Statistics of 2004 shows that 99.8 % of federal prison sentences for drug offenses were for drug trafficking.[6] *Drug Possession Offenders in USA State Prisons 2004*: Drug possession 6%, crimes involving marijuana 1.4%, marijuana only drug offenders; no prior sentences .40%, marijuana possession only .30%, marijuana only possession no prior sentences 0.10%.[6]

According to the Bureau of Justice Statistics report of 2008; 80% of State inmates were in prison for crimes other than drug offenses and only 0.3% were imprisoned for possession of marijuana.[7] Those in prison for possession are often a result of plea bargaining.[8] In the federal prison system, only 1.6% were sentenced by the federal courts for possession of marijuana. Of those federal inmates, the median amount of marijuana possession was 155 pounds.[9]

"Under our current laws few offenders are in prison for marijuana possession. No more than two-tenths of one percent (0.2%) of federal inmates are locked up for marijuana possession and, among state prisoners, only one-tenth of one percent (0.1%) are in for marijuana possession without a prior record. Predictably, most of these prisoners were charged with probation or parole violations or with possession of wholesale quantities where intent to distribute could not be proved."[10] —David G. Evans, Esq.

In Colorado in 2010, only 1% of court commitments to prison in 2010 involved marijuana charges. There were more court commitments to prison for traffic-related offences as for all marijuana offences.[10]

WHO IS IN PRISON FOR MARIJUANA POSSESSION IN CANADA? *The nature and extent of marijuana possession in British Columbia,* produced by the Centre for Public Safety and Research Justice Research Justice Institute in 2013 shows, marijuana possession only cases cleared by a charge (solved by) in 2011: 249 cases with 169 proceeding to court, 42 convicted, and 7 resulted in a custody sentence. Of the 7 that resulted in a custody sentence, 4 received one day in jail terms, 2 received

7 day jail terms, and 1 received a 14 day jail term.

The typical history of those convicted; 90% had a prior criminal history, with the average length of criminal history being 12 years; prior drug offenses 64%, prior criminal driving offenses 30%, prior property offenses 75%, prior violent offenses 64%, of those with ten or more prior offenses amounted to 57%.[11]

A study by the US Department of Justice showed that 35% of inmates reported they were under the influence of drugs at the time they committed their crime. Marijuana and hashish were cited as the most frequently used at the time of the crime."[12]

"Marijuana is a factor in over 50% of crimes committed (ADAMII report). 59% of arrestees in Sacramento test positive for marijuana. Sacramento also ranks number 1 in the nation for an increase in violent crime, undoubtedly related to the 30 licensed dispensaries selling pot." —Roger Morgan, *Take Back America Campaign*

A study published in the *International Journal of Addiction*, involving interviews with 268 inmates in New York prison for homicide, revealed that 70% had used marijuana within twenty four hours of committing the crime and felt they experienced some effect from the drug at the time of the crime.[13] Twenty-five percent felt the homicide was related to their use of marijuana before the crime.[13]

In Denver, over 50% of those arrested admitted to being regular marijuana users.[14] Urine tests were positive for marijuana among 40% of adult males arrested.[14]

DECRIMINALIZATION In September 2010, Governor Arnold Schwarzenegger signed *California State Assembly Bill 1449 (AB 1449)* into law. This new law reduced the sanction for possessing less than one ounce of marijuana from a misdemeanor to an infraction, legally the equivalent of a parking ticket. This essentially decriminalized the personal consumption of up to one ounce of marijuana. In the State of California arrests for simple possession, of one ounce, is an infraction with a $100 non-escalating fine.

Oregon was the first state to decriminalize possession of small amounts in 1973. Marijuana decriminalization, as of 2017, was the law in thirteen states.

In 2014, under the Conservative government lead by Prime Minister Stephen Harper, there were ongoing discussion between the Canadian Minister of Justice, Peter Mackay, law enforcement agencies and the legal sector over a proposal to move to a ticketing offense for small amounts of marijuana possession.[15]

The Canadian Police Chiefs voted in favor of a resolution in August of 2014: "There are instances when having an alternative to attending (criminal) court would be beneficial....There are circumstances where a formal charge for simple possession is appropriate, such as getting caught with a joint while driving, or when individuals caught have existing criminal records."[16]

University of Ottawa law professor Graham Mayeda outlined to *CBC News* the different ways the federal government could introduce new legislation without decriminalizing marijuana possession.[17] He told the media that the government could retain simple possession of marijuana as a criminal offence, under the *Controlled Drugs and Substances Act*, but they could change the law by reducing the penalty; a monetary fine rather than jail time could be put forward; adding that to move the offence out of the *Criminal Code*, would move legal enforcement from federal to provincial jurisdictions.[17]

In 2012, Canada brought in changes to drug charges under the *Safe Streets and Communities Act*. The changes included increasing minimum jail time to two years for individuals found to be guilty of trafficking near a school. Under the *Controlled Drug and Substances Act of the Criminal Code of Canada*, a person found guilty of possession, can be sentenced to jail time, and first time offenders can be fined up to $1,000 or face six months in jail. Discretionary power rests with individual law enforcement agencies and regional governments.

The *CBC* on August 19, 2014 printed a response to the suggestion of decriminalization possibly being introduced in Canada from a representative of the NORML Women's Alliance of Canada which revealed a concern that such a move could "placate" people into concluding the marijuana problem was solved.[18]

Ticketing could prove to be a beneficial tool in reducing use by youth and better facilitate early parental involvement in the use of drugs by their children. The immediacy of a penalty has been shown to be particularly effective in reducing infractions by youth.[19]

A key point of contention for the pot activists has been the idea that the real harm from the use of marijuana comes not from the plant itself but from the penalties placed on young "offenders", including a ruined career, a thwarted education and the hardship of being denied travel across international borders.[20,21,22] There are measures in place to protect youth from being burdened with criminal records for committing offences in both Canada and the United States.

The Youth Criminal Justice Act in Canada protects the privacy of young people who are accused or found guilty of a crime by keeping their identity and other personal information confidential with access only by certain people including law enforcement, legal professionals, parents or guardians and victims. There are some variations to this protection such as the offender reoffending during the "access period". Once the access period has passed the records are sealed or destroyed.

Dr. Harold Kalant wrote a commentary, *A critique of cannabis legalization proposals in Canada*, for the *International Journal of Drug Policy* (April 27 2016), in response to the CAMH document—*Cannabis Policy Framework* (Crepault, 2014).[23, 24] Dr. Kalant referenced a specific CAMH statement; "Around 60,000 Canadians are arrested for simple possession of cannabis every year."[23, 24] Statistics Canada is cited as the source of the data. Dr. Kalant makes the argument, that the authors of the CAMH paper do not clarify their statement with the fact that Statistics Canada records all cannabis incidents, regardless of whether cannabis possession is the principal object of the incident or only a minor accompaniment to other charges, and goes on to further explain that the statistics give no indications of the outcomes.[23]

Dr. Kalant points to the data from Statistics Canada that shows that 699,000 Canadians have criminal records due to a conviction of marijuana possession but that many of these convictions occurred decades ago and that there has been a diversion of cases at an increasing frequency from the justice system to that of health care. Pardons have been available.[23]

PROTECTION FOR MINORS For over a century, The United States has had special provisions in place for the protection of minors found guilty of crimes, as individual states have established separate court systems for handling juveniles charged with offenses. In most states delinquency is defined as the commission of an act by a child who is under the age of 18, most states also allow youth to remain under the supervision of the juvenile court until age 21. Records are often confidential, protecting children from carrying the burden of their delinquent activity into adulthood. Juvenile records in most jurisdictions are not automatically sealed or expunged.

"Juvenile crime has steadily decreased since the early 1990's. However, when juvenile crime rates rose nationwide in the late 1980's and early 1990's, states adopted 'get-tough' policies for crimes, depriving certain youth of the juvenile justice system's protections."[24] —Juvenile Law Center

Decriminalization typically means no arrest, no risk of incarceration, or criminal record for the first-time possession of a small amount of marijuana for personal consumption. Decriminalization is a legal discussion over what penalties fit a crime or infraction. Changes can be made to the way marijuana use is sanctioned without moving to full scale legalization and providing for commercialization.

Under Canadian law "drug courts" could be a feasible option. Under the Canadian criminal justice system, modelled after that of the United Kingdom, no individual can be compelled to go to a police station except by order of arrest. Moving to a "drug court" program would require the continued involvement of the criminal justice system in drug enforcement even if the court served to caution versus charge people who were brought before them.

Eleven US states decriminalized minor personal possession of marijuana between 1973 and 1978.[26] The next state to decriminalize marijuana was Nevada in 2001.

In Colorado if an individual, who is under the age of 21, is caught with retail marijuana they could be given a *Minor in Possession Charge*, which could result in a fine, a driver's license suspension, and misdemeanor or felony charges. For a first offense the penalty can be a fine of $100, or a court order to complete a substance abuse education program, and possibly a driver's license suspension. A second offense includes the same and it is also possible that the individual will be have to submit to an Office of Behavioral Health for a substance abuse assessment and complete any treatment that is recommended by the assessment, and in addition they may be ordered to perform up to 24 hours of public service. On a third offense the fine is increased to $250.00 and a court order to submit to the assessment and complete treatment, and perform up to 36 hours of public service.

"Marijuana charges, including Minor in Possession (MIP) charges, can result in the loss of federal financial aid for college, including: *Perkins Loans, Pell Grants, Supplemental Educational Opportunity Grants, PLUS Loans*, and *Work-Study Programs*."[27] —Colorado PHE 2017.

THE ROCKEFELLER DRUG LAWS "The study of history raises a vital question here: can we preserve and integrate a healthier lifestyle without going so far in our desire to reform that a backlash will undercut and sweep away the advances that have been made in public health?...Moreover, insistence on dramatic change obscures real but more gradual progress, and can provide exaggerated responses and create a false sense of defeat. Drug policy remains vulnerable to the forces of frustration and fatigue."[28] —Dr. David Musto

In 1960, 169 federal marijuana violations were recorded (Solomon 1966). By 1970 the number had increased to 190,000; 421,000 by 1973; 446,000 in 1974 and stayed above 400,000 into the mid 1980s (Slaughter, 1988).[29]

Nelson A. Rockefeller (1908–1979) was the governor of the state of New York from 1958 to 1973. In 1974, he was appointed Vice President by President Gerald Ford after Nixon left the White House. During his term, as the Governor of New York, Rockefeller created the Narcotic Addiction and Control Commission in 1967, in response to escalating drug use and the ensuing problems of addiction.

In the early 1970s, New York City was experiencing a heroin epidemic and a high homicide rate. The Governor decided to radically change course on his approach to the issue of drug prevention and control. He changed from viewing the problem as primarily a social problem and pivoted to support increasing the penalties for drug trafficking. His change of strategy, considered to have been influenced by the Japanese tough on crime and drugs approach, found support in the New York legislature.[30] The State's own tough on drug statures would come to be known as *Rockefeller Drug Laws*.

"I have one goal and one objective, and that is to stop the pushing of drugs and to protect the innocent victim," said Governor Rockefeller.[31] At a press conference in January of 1973, the Governor called for mandatory prison sentences of 15 years to life for drug dealing and addicts, including those caught with small amounts of marijuana, cocaine or heroin.[31] Mandatory sentences had been introduced in 1951, had been abolished in 1950, and then were re-introduced as public sentiment and political power reacted to the problem of drug use.

Drug offenders, as a percentage of New York's prison population, surged from 11% in 1973 to a peak of 35% in 1994, according to the state's Corrections Department.[32] Following the example set in 1973 by New York other states began to enact laws to deal with their own drug problems. By 1983, 49 states had provisions for mandatory minimum sentences for offenses.

By the mid-1980s, there was support for reducing drug supply and demand, under the Ronald Reagan administration. The crack epidemic and the fear of HIV/Aids were factors in driving drug control measures, along with a growing concern over violent drug crimes.

Stricter mandatory minimum sentencing laws, which resulted in new tougher laws came in 1984, 1986, 1988.[31] In 1986, the Reagan Administration passed a law requiring federal judges to give fixed sentences to drug offenders based on variables, including the amount of drug products seized and the presence of firearms.

Between 1980 and 1993 the number of arrests for drug offenses, made by State and local police, doubled.[32] The total of arrest for 1980 were dominated by marijuana related charges. However, the increase in the drug arrests from 1983 onward were mostly for opium and cocaine and not marijuana.[33] The high point for arrests for marijuana had been in 1982. Of the felony convictions in state courts in 1992, 1.8% involved marijuana.[33]

Over the period of 1980-1992, there was a 346% increase in the number of federal defendants sentenced to prison in U.S. District Courts for drug offenses, compared to a 71% increase for non-drug offenses.[33]

A thorough and very informative document is that of *Cannabis Use in the United States Implications for Policy* by Lana D. Harrison, Michael Backenheimer and James A. Inciardi. A particular interesting set of numbers that they refer to are for the outcomes of the defendants in the U.S. District Courts for 1992. The data shows that there were 5,657 marijuana defendants before the courts in respect to disposition of a case of which: 814 of these were dismissed by the court, 15 were acquitted by the court, and 88 were acquitted by a jury. Of the defendants convicted by the court, the 4,283 entered a plea of guilty, 2 defendants pled nolo contendere, 34 were convicted by the court and 421 were convicted by a jury (Maquire and Pastore, 1994).[34]

A study commissioned by Attorney General Janet Reno in 1993 concluded that more than one-fifth of the federal prison population consists of low-level drug offenders, defined as persons convicted of drug crimes who have no prior prison time, no current or prior violence in their records, and no involvement in sophisticated criminal activity.[35] In reviewing this statement it is relevant to consider the duration of the sentence and the length of prison stay and the wide-spread practise of plea bargaining.

In 2004, Governor George Pataki of New York, signed the *Drug Law Reform Act*, a move that significantly changed *The Rockefeller Laws* sentencing guidelines. The mandatory minimum was lessened to 8 to 20 years and those convicted of serious offenses were permitted to apply for lighter sentences.

Ongoing drug policies discussions would do well to disassociate from those who seek retribution for policies implemented in the past, policies that may be viewed as overly punitive and excessive and to separate fact from fiction.

"I was a prosecutor for several years, and the facts are quite different. Smoking pot has actually been "de facto" legalized across the U.S. The police look the other way, even if a neighbor rats on someone....

Regardless of one's position on drug legalization, stop saying that people are serving time behind bars for marijuana possession. You just look silly."[36] —Rachel Alexander (2013)

16. Playing Tough

BIG MARIJUANA TRASHES DEMOCRATIC PROCESS. *—The Gazette.* The editorial board of *The Gazette,* in Colorado Springs, published the following editorial on July 8, 2016: *"Those who despise Big Tobacco's notorious electioneering ain't seen nothing yet. Big Tobacco 2.0, aka Big Marijuana, can negate Colorado's grassroots petition process—which helped establish the industry:* When Colorado voters legalized marijuana, they meant well. They wanted a safe trade, regulated like alcohol. They ended up with a system of, by and for Big Marijuana. It is a racket in which the will of voters gets quashed before votes are cast. Any doubt about Big Marijuana's disregard for Colorado's desire for good regulation will disappear with a new revelation: the industry bought away the public's chance to vote.

That's right. Big Marijuana bought away a proposed vote on regulations in Colorado, where we vote on fixing potholes. At issue is proposed ballot initiative *139,* written to give voters a few reasonable options to improve regulation of recreational pot sales. The measure proposed no changes for medical marijuana. On recreational sales, it would have:

Required child-resistant packaging, as we have for aspirin

and ibuprofen. Put health warnings on marijuana labels. Restricted product THC potency to 16 percent, even though THC occurs naturally at only .2 to .5 percent in cannabis. *Initiative 139* was so reasonable, so in line with the intentions of voters who legalized pot, recent polling showed 80 percent support among registered voters.

Big Marijuana opposes *139* because the industry wants to do as it pleases. It views potency restrictions, which would keep Colorado's pot products among the more potent in the world, as a sales barrier. Big Marijuana doesn't want the nuisance of labeling requirements and child-resistant packaging.

Knowing *139* was likely to pass, Big Marijuana sued to keep it off the ballot. The suit stalled efforts to raise money and recruit voluntary signature gatherers. When the Colorado Supreme Court ruled in defense of letting voters decide, Big Marijuana's anti-*139* campaign paid Colorado's major signature firms to avoid gathering signatures for the pro-*139* campaign. 'They were offering $75,000 to $200,000 depending on size of each company, to get contracts that say they will not gather signatures for this ballot measure,' said attorney and former Colorado House Speaker Frank McNulty, passing along information an anti-*139* consultant shared with him.

As Big Marijuana paid for anti-petition contracts, the price of collecting signatures rose. Advocates of *139* responded by raising more money. Former lawmaker Patrick Kennedy, son of former Sen. Ted Kennedy, swooped in to help with a last-ditch fundraising effort this week that boosted the *139* war chest to nearly $800,000. Just when the campaign planned to hire an Arizona-based firm to gather signatures, Big Marijuana paid the company off.

'The narrative of the marijuana industry has been 'don't meddle with our business, because the voters have spoken and the will of the voters is sacred. This is a democracy'. Then we have a genuine democratic effort to improve recreational marijuana regulation, and the industry shuts down democracy with big money and a bag of dirty tricks,' said Ben Cort, a member of the board of directors of Smart Approaches to Marijuana. 'It became clear. No matter how much money we raised, and who we tried to hire, they were going to prevent voters from having any say.'

It is a sad day when an industry's lawyers can buy away the people's opportunity to petition for a vote, even after the state's highest court defended the process. Big Marijuana stopped *139* by stomping on Colorado voters—the people who legalized their industry—as if their will should no longer count. Big Marijuana is officially corrupt."[1]

OHIO AND MARIJUANA Ohio was scheduled to vote on legalization in the November 2015 election. The proposed ballot initiative if successful would have made marijuana legal for adults 21+ years of age and have limited the number of growers to ten. The organization behind the initiative was called *Responsible OH*. *Responsible OH* raised $21.2 million, from 10 investment groups, to bring legalization to the Ohio ballot.[3]

The initiative also wanted voters to permit adults to grow four plants and have provided medical marijuana at cost, along with 1,000 retail and manufacturing licenses for commercialization. Ohio defeated *Responsible OH*.

OREGON AND MARIJUANA In Oregon, the Drug Policy Alliance of New York City and the Marijuana Policy Project of Washington DC, along with proponents raised $570,000 in 2012 to the opponent $71,000 for *New Approach Oregon*.[3] Oregon voters rejected *Measure 80* in 2012. If passed the measure would have allowed adults over the age of 21 to possess an unlimited supply of marijuana and given an industry-dominated board permission to regulate sales.

In 2014, pro-marijuana supporters pumped at least $14.4 million into the Oregon campaign versus an approximate $324,000 in opposition.[3] For Ballot Measure 91 to legalize recreational marijuana in Oregon three billionaires spent $5,965,410 and only $118,000 came from in-state individual proponents.[3] The state of Oregon, in November 2014, voted to legally permit the sale and consumption of recreational cannabis. The initiative provisions gave users the right to possess a half pound of marijuana at a time, plus 4 plants, an amount 8 times the amount legally allowed in Colorado, Washington or Alaska.

COLORADO CAMPAIGN "Youth past-month marijuana use increased 20% in the two years (2013/2014) since Colorado legalized recreational marijuana, compared to the two-year average prior to legalization (2011/2012). Nationally, youth past-month marijuana use declined 4% during the same time. The latest 2013/2014 results, show that Colorado youth ranked #1 in the nation for past-month marijuana use, up from #4 in 2011/2012, and #14 in 2005/2006. Colorado youth past-month marijuana use for 2013/2014 was 74% higher than the national average compared to 39% higher in 2011/2012.

College-age past-month marijuana use increased 17% in the two-year average (2013/2014) since Colorado legalized recreational marijuana, compared to the two-year average prior to legalization (2011/2012).

Nationally college-age past month marijuana use increased 2% during the same time. The latest 2013/2014 results show Colorado college-age adults ranked #1 in the nation for past-month marijuana use, up from #3 in 2011/2012 and #8 in 2005/2006. Colorado college-age past-month marijuana use for 2013/2014 was 62% higher than the national average, compared to 42% higher in 2011/2012.

Adult past-month marijuana use increased 63% in the two year average (2013/2014) since Colorado legalized recreational marijuana, compared to the two-year average prior to legalization (2011/2012). Nationally, adult past-month marijuana use increased 21% during the same time.

The latest 2013/2014 results show Colorado adults ranked #1 in the nation for past-month marijuana use, up from #7 in 2011/2012 and #8 in 2005/2006. Colorado adult past-month marijuana use for 2013/2014, was 104% higher than the national average compared to 51% higher in 2011/2012.

The national rate for past-month marijuana use by youth, for ages 12 to 17 for the 2013/2014 period, stood at 7.22%;compared to Colorado at 12.56%,Vermont at 11.40%, Oregon at 10.19%, Washington at 10.06%, Maine at 9.90%, Alaska at 9.19%, Massachusetts at 8.88% and California standing at 8.74%."[4] —RMHIDTA 2016

CBS News in January of 2017, reported on a study of marijuana use by teenagers in Washington and Colorado. The report found in Washington State, that since 2012, marijuana use among eighth graders had increased by 2%, and 4.1% for tenth graders but in Colorado legalization had resulted in no impact on marijuana use by teenagers.[5]

Data provided from The US Department of Health and Human Services, the *National Survey on Drug Use and Health*, and *The US Monitoring the Future Study*, all show an increase in kids using marijuana in Colorado after legalization.[4,5,6,7]

Letter of March 10, 2017 to Governor Hickenlooper: "We are a group of scientists from Harvard University and other institutions acutely concerned about the impact of marijuana on youth, and among drivers, employees, parents, and other members of society.

We understand your continued skepticism with regards to "recreational" marijuana legalization, but are concerned about recent statements you made on national television regarding youth marijuana use in Colorado. In response to a question about marijuana asked by Chuck Todd on *Meet the Press* (February 26, 2017), you replied that there was no increase in teenage use and that the black market was shrinking.

However, data we have reviewed points us toward a very different conclusion. The only representative sample of teens ever conducted in Colorado, the *National Survey on Drug Use and Health* (*NSDUH*), shows that Colorado now leads the nation among 12 to 17-year-olds in (A) last-year marijuana use, (B) last-month marijuana use, and (C) the percentage of people who try marijuana for the first time during that period ("first use").

You may have been referencing press summaries of the *Healthy Kids Colorado Survey* (*HKCS*). Unlike the *NSDUH*, however, that study is not a reliable or representative indicator. *HKCS* fails to include data from Colorado's second and third-most-populous counties (Jefferson and Douglas Counties), as well as El Paso County. It also omits kids who

are not in school and raises the threshold for statistical significance to the point that it disguises changes from year to year.
For these reasons, the Centers for Disease Control refuses to
include *HKCS* in its *Youth Behavior Risk Survey* (*YRBS*).

Even taking *HKCS* into account, youth use has risen state-
wide since legalization at about the same rate tobacco use has
fallen in that same timeframe. The increase since 2013 halted
a four-year trend of declining marijuana use; the turning point
occurred exactly when the state legalized pot. Additionally,
swings in youth use per *HKCS* are quite large in some counties where pot shops are prevalent. For instance, the Summit/
Eagle/Vail area reported a 90% increase in use among high
school seniors in the last two years, and the NW Steamboat/
Craig region showed a 58% increase in the same timeframe.

With respect to the black market for marijuana, your own
Attorney General Cynthia Coffman said, 'The criminals are still
selling on the black market. ...We have plenty of cartel activity in
Colorado (and) plenty of illegal activity that has not decreased at
all.' Indeed, organized crime filings have skyrocketed in Colorado.
The state had one such filing in 2007 and by 2015, it had 40.

That surge coincides precisely with the state's commercialization of medical marijuana in 2009, and legalization
of non-medical marijuana in 2012. Lt. Mark Comte of the
Colorado Springs Police Vice and Narcotics Unit similarly
commented that legalization 'has done nothing more than
enhance the opportunity for the black market.' A federal law
enforcement official also characterized Colorado as 'the black
market for the rest of the country,' a statement supported
by the sharp increase in seizures of marijuana mailed out of
Colorado since legalization.

Moreover, the legalization of pot in Colorado appears to have opened the door for Mexican cartel operations in the heart of the United States. A representative of the Colorado Attorney General's office noted in 2016 that legalization "has inadvertently helped fuel the business of Mexican drug cartels...cartels are now trading drugs like heroin for marijuana, and the trade has since opened the door to drug and human trafficking."

Similarly, the Drug Enforcement Administration reported that 'since 2014, there has been a noticeable increase in organized networks of sophisticated residential (marijuana) grows in Colorado that are orchestrated and operated by drug trafficking organizations.' The mayor of Colorado Springs, John Suthers, agreed, stating that 'Mexican cartels are no longer sending marijuana into Colorado, they're now growing it in Colorado and sending it back to Mexico and every place elseix,' hiding in plain sight among legal operations. As you can see, there are serious problems with suggesting that legalizing marijuana has been a positive development for public health, youth use, and law enforcement.

Further, marijuana-involved traffic fatalities, poison control calls, emergency room visits, and treatment center utilization have all increased in Colorado since legalization. We hope that you will clear the air and correct the record in your next media appearance." —Sincerely, **Stuart Gitlow**, M.D., M.P.H., M.B.A. Executive Director Annenberg Physician Training Program in Addictive Disease, **Sharon Levy**, M.D., M.P.H. Associate Professor of Pediatrics, Harvard Medical School Director, Adolescent Substance Abuse Program Boston Children's Hospital **Paula D. Riggs**, M.D., M.A. Director, Division of Substance Dependence, Department of Psychiatry

University of Colorado School of Medicine, **Hoover Adger**, M.D., M.P.H. Professor of Pediatrics, Johns Hopkins University, **Sion Harris**, PhD, CPH Assistant Professor of Pediatrics, Harvard University Co-Director, Boston Children's Hospital Center for Adolescent Substance Abuse Research, **Judge Arthur L. Burnett, Sr.** (Ret.) Executive Director, National African American Drug Policy Coalition, **Christian Thurstone**, M.D. Associate Professor, Psychiatry, University of Colorado Past President, Colorado Child and Adolescent Psychiatric Society, **Howard C. Samuels**, Psy.D., Founder of The Hills Treatment Center, **Roneet Lev**, M.D. Director of Operations, Scripps Mercy Emergency Department Emergency Medicine Former President, California Chapter, American College of Emergency Physicians.[8]

A *Monitoring the Future* survey of students in grades 8, 10 and 12, reported 10% of high school students who would otherwise be at low risk for habitual pot smoking say that they would use marijuana if it were legal.[9] "Low risk" was defined by the researchers as kids who didn't smoke cigarettes, have strong religious beliefs, and have no friends who smoke marijuana products.[9]

Colorado child welfare cases, involving drug use by a parent or foster parent, went up by about 2 percentage points from 2013 to 2015, although there was a decline in the total number of new child welfare cases.[10] Colorado child welfare workers intervene when a newborn tests positive for marijuana, when a child has ingested marijuana, or when it is determined that a parent or caregiver's use of marijuana products poses harm to a child's welfare.[10]

At a Joint Budget Committee meeting in December of 2016

staff suggested that county child welfare departments tap into money from the state's marijuana tax cash fund. Child welfare caseloads had increased since marijuana legalization in the State of Colorado, specifically cases related to child marijuana exposure, reported budget staff officers.[11] "The precise impact of marijuana on child abuse and neglect cases is unknown. The state child welfare department's computer system does not track drug-specific information, although that will change next year."[10] —Jennifer Brown, reporter, *Denver Post*

A pediatrician and medical director of the newborn intensive-care unit of Pueblo Colorado's Saint Mary Corwin Medical Center, told *60 Minutes*, that in the first nine months of 2016 the numbers of babies born testing positive for THC was about 15% higher than the year before at the medical center. "I try to explain to them (new mothers) that even though you're not smoking very much, the baby is getting seven times more than you're taking and that there's—this drug has been shown to cause harm in developing brains."[12,13] —Dr. Stephen Simerville, *The Pot Vote*, CBS (2016)

"Heavy users drive almost 70% of total marijuana demand, and the prevalence of heavy users in Colorado is higher than the national average. According to the *National Survey on Drug Use and Health*, 23% of the user population in Colorado consumes near daily, compared with a 17% share nationwide. The second highest user cohort is also larger, with a 9% share in Colorado, compared to a 6 percent share nationwide."[14] —Colorado Department of Revenue

17. The Insult

Mason Tvert, an American marijuana activist, in 2015 told *CBS News* (Denver, Colorado) that there was no evidence to link the use of marijuana with suicide.[1]

2013 data from the *Vermont's Youth Risk Behavior Survey* shows a striking correspondence between suicide attempts and the rate of marijuana use, consistent with larger, better controlled studies on suicide.[2]

About 15% of all users and a much higher percentage of heavy users will experience psychotic symptoms.[3]

Long Lasting Effects of Chronic Heavy Cannabis Abuse, published in March, 2017 in the *American Journal on Addictions* relates that 40% of the participants in a study experienced auditory hallucinations, and 54% experienced dilutions. That these symptoms persisted three months after the use of marijuana use the research scientists called a "remarkable" finding.[4]

Kevin Reed, the founder and president of *The Green Cross*, a medical marijuana dispensary in San Francisco, told staff writer Kurtis Alexander of the *San Francisco Chronicle*: "The context disappears with legalization," he said. "It just becomes getting high." "It's going to be a different world," he added: "It's not really the world I signed up for. But I'm going to take the ride."[5] A study of California medical marijuana patients found that the average user was a 32-year old white male, with a history of alcohol and substance abuse, and no history of a life-threatening medical condition.[6]

THE INTERVIEWS The executive director of the Drug Policy Alliance, told the *Huffington Post* that he credits his organization as the driving force behind legalizing marijuana, first for medical use and then for recreational use. He says legalization is a policy grounded in science, compassion, health, and human rights.[7] Drug Policy Alliance Website lists ten facts about marijuana, including a statement that long-term marijuana smoking is not associated with an elevated cancer risk.[7]

Zach Walsh, a psychology professor at the University of British Columbia, with a focus on marijuana research, when asked in an interview about marijuana dependency replied: "It's not the kind of thing that if they wanted to do it, they'd need to engage in intensive psycho-behavioral reorganization of their lives to conquer the addiction. There is a modest dependence profile of cannabis, less profound than with caffeine."[8]

DOWNPLAYING THE RISKS "How much is a government going to save because they don't have to incarcerate somebody because they have six pot plants? Because we don't have to arrange undercover officers to arrange for deals for something that doesn't hurt us."[9] —John Moore, guest on *CBC News-The National* (2015)

"As long as you don't get caught with cannabis, it's not going to do you any harm. The criminalisation around cannabis is way more harmful than anything else that can happen with it. Tobacco kills older people, alcohol kills younger people, cannabis doesn't kill anyone," said David Nutt, Ph.D.[10]

The Journal of the American Heart Association in 2014, reported: "Marijuana use may result in cardiovascular-related complications—even death—among young and middle-aged adults, according to a French study reporting.[11] Cannabis use can lead to severe cardiovascular problems and sudden death, not only in people at increased cardiovascular risk, but also in young people without any medical history or risk factors.[11]

On March 29, 2017, a study from McMaster University and St. Joseph's Healthcare in Canada showed cannabis use as a predictor for continued opioid use by those seeking treatment with methadone.[12] The researchers found that for women undergoing methadone treatment, those that also use marijuana products were 82% more likely to continue with using opioids. Of those enrolled in methadone treatment therapy approximately 60% of men and 44% of women report they also use marijuana products.[12]

PREGNANCY Some of the US states, who have legalized medipot, are failing to pass laws that address giving proper notice to consumers regarding pregnancy and marijuana harms.

The Arizona Department of Health Services is setting a good example by adopting warnings of potential risks related to medical marijuana and pregnancy. The rules require each certifying physician to address the potential dangers to fetuses caused by smoking or ingesting marijuana while pregnant or to infants while breastfeeding and the risk of being reported to the Department of Child Safety.[13] Arizona pot retailers in 2016 were required to post warnings.

An article written by Paul Armentano, *Breathe, Push, Puff? Pot Use and Pregnancy*: A *Review of the Literature (2009)*, discussed survey data from the journal, *Complementary Therapies in Clinical Practice,* that showed of 84 surveyed women 36 of the women said that they had used cannabis intermittently during their pregnancy to treat symptoms of vomiting, nausea, and appetite loss.[14] The article concluded that it could be argued that the pre-natal and post-natal dangers posed by maternal pot use, particularly for moderate use, were rather minimal and added that this was the case, especially when compared to inutero exposure to the alcohol and tobacco.[14]

Marijuana is the most frequently used illicit drug during pregnancy in both Canada and the United States.[15] Based on data from the *National Survey on Drug Use and Health* for the years 2011/2012, in the United States, 5.2% of pregnant women, ages 15-44, reported past-month cannabis use, slightly higher than the number using from 2009/2010 (3.6%).[16] The use of cannabis was reportedly highest during the first trimester (10.7%), as compared to the second (2.8%), and third (2.3%) trimester.[17]

At least half of all pregnancies in North America are unplanned.[18] Nearly 11% of Canadian women of childbearing age (15–44 years) reported past-year use of cannabis in 2011 reported Health Canada.[19] These conditions clearly establish that there is potential risk for offspring.

The Colorado report, *Monitoring Changes in Marijuana Use Patterns 2017,* reported on the percentage of women who were using marijuana while pregnant: women ages 20-24 13%, ages 25-34 4%, ages 35 and older 3%.[20] Women with less than a grade 12 education used marijuana while pregnant 16% of the time, in comparison to 4% those with some college credits. Approximately 5% of mothers, who were breast-feeding their infants, were using marijuana. Marijuana products were used in 4% of intended pregnancies and 9% of unintended. Six percentage of all new mothers in Colorado told researchers that they had used marijuana during pregnancy, 13% reported they had used alcohol, and 6% had used tobacco products.[20]

Marijuana use among pregnant women rose 62% between 2002 and 2014, according to findings of a study published in the December 2016 issue of the *Journal of the American Medical Association*.[21]

Writing in their 1997 book, *Marijuana Myths, Marijuana Facts: A Review of the Scientific Evidence* (The Lindesmith Center), Drs. John M. Morgan and Lynn Zimmer asserted that marijuana had no reliable impact on birth size, or length of gestation, nor on the occurrence of physical abnormalities among infants. The authors cite large-scale surveys that they claim "appear" to back up their conclusions.[22]

The online magazine, *Cannabis Culture*, discusses marijuana use in pregnancy, for relief of nausea, loss of appetite and to help get emotions under control, and claim that most studies say cannabis is perfectly safe during pregnancy, and add that the topic is "controversial."[23]

LONG TERM CONSEQUENCES   Smoking marijuana during pregnancy has been shown to decrease a baby's birth weight, most likely due to the effects of carbon monoxide on the developing fetus.[24] The long term consequences may be far more damaging than the short term relief of symptoms. Marijuana crosses the placental barrier and has effects on the newborn baby. The growing evidence for a negative impact of prenatal cannabis exposure originates from three longitudinal studies worldwide.[24, 25, 26] Two of the studies have tested children for the longest period of time, and their findings show neurocognitive challenges in the areas of short-term memory, as well as verbal outcomes, aspects of attention, impulsivity and abstract visual skill performance.[25] These deficits appear after age 3 and continue into young adulthood.

Most significantly, at 6 years of age, children exposed prenatally to marijuana showed more impulsive and hyperactive behavior. This continued into adolescence and was accompanied by problems in abstract and visual reasoning, as well as visuo-perceptual functioning.[25]

These are the types of skills required to perform "top down processing", such as good decision making, organizing behavior, setting goals and putting into action a plan to accomplish the goals. Each of these cognitive processes can be grouped under the umbrella term of executive functioning. Executive functioning is required for success in life, including schooling, interaction, relationships and work life. Struggles can occur in these facets when executive functions are compromised, something that can occur with prenatal marijuana exposure.

A growing body of evidence suggests that marijuana use during pregnancy can negatively impact pre-natal and postnatal development. Marijuana use, particularly heavy use, during pregnancy can result in an increased likelihood of distorted facial features compared to *Fetal Alcohol Syndrome* babies, deficits in memory, verbal and perceptual skills, and verbal and visual reasoning, beginning at age three or four.[27]

Impaired performance in reasoning and short term memory

have been observed at age six onwards, and deficits in reading, spelling and achievement, have been observed at around nine years of age.[26]

Medical complications for the mother and child can arise from using illicit drugs during pregnancy. These negative outcomes include a pregnancy loss, a detached placenta, fetal growth restrictions, blood clots, heightened blood pressure, intrauterine death, preterm labour and hemorrhaging following labour. In utero, a fetus can become dependent on drugs that are transmitted through the blood stream and cross the placenta.[28]

The March of Dimes discusses pregnancy and marijuana on their website and alerts women that if marijuana is smoked during pregnancy, the chances of stillbirth are twice as likely.[29]

In 2016, American entertainer Whoopi Goldberg lent her name and support to a marijuana for medi-pot company—Maya & Whoopi. The company was launching a line of products designed to provide relief from menstrual cramps.[30] Women who begin using marijuana during their reproductive years may be unable to stop during a pregnancy.

WARNING TO PARENTS-TO-BE   Cannabinoids are psychoactive, all are bioactive. These chemicals may remain in the body's fatty tissues for extensive periods of times with unknown consequences. THC is excreted into human breast milk and affects quality and quantity of this important source of nutrition. THC can accumulate in human breast milk to high concentrations, and infants exposed to marijuana, passed through their mother's milk, will excrete THC in their urine for two to three weeks.[31] Studies conducted on animals show that marijuana can inhibit lactation by inhibiting prolactin production.[32]

Marijuana products can produce sedation and growth delay in infant and studies have demonstrated that for babies exposed to marijuana through breast feeding may have trouble with sucking.[33]

An important phase of brain growth occurs during a baby's first months of life and THC could theoretically alter brain cells metabolism. There are no studies on the long-term effects of THC exposure through breast milk on a developing infant but a study is currently underway in Colorado.[34]

Dr. Steven Simerville, the medical director of the newborn intensive care unit at St. Mary-Corwin Medical Center in Pueblo, Colorado warns: "What I'm seeing in our nursery is a dramatic increase in babies who test positive for marijuana. The interesting thing for me is the number of mothers who use marijuana and want to breast feed. They don't believe marijuana is harmful."[35] —The Denver Post

A calculation of the time it takes from the beginning of drinking until clearance of alcohol from breast milk for women can be calculated, the same cannot be said at this time for marijuana. Alcohol is water soluble whereas marijuana is fat soluble and is excreted from the human body very differently.

"Alcohol consumed by the mother passes into her bloodstream and her breast milk. Alcohol levels in the breast milk are similar to the blood alcohol levels of the mother at the time of feeding. Alcohol leaves the body as it is metabolized. A breast-feeding infant is exposed to a very small amount of the alcohol the mother drinks, but infants detoxify alcohol in their first weeks of life at half the rate of adults. Alcohol is not stored in the breast milk and passed to the infant at a later feeding.... Excessive or daily intake of alcohol is not recommended for

any mother due to issues of impairment of care and the risk of fetal alcohol spectrum disorder for a subsequent pregnancy."[36]
—*Motherisk*

For a 40.8-kg (90-lb) woman who consumed three drinks in 1 hour, it would take 8 hours, 30 minutes for there to be no alcohol in her breast milk. For a 63.5-kg (140-lb) woman drinking four beers starting at 8:00 pm, it would take 9 hours, 17 minutes for there to be no alcohol in her breast milk (i.e., until 5:17 am). *1 drink = 340 g 319 (12 oz.) of 5% beer, or 141.75 g (5 oz.) of 11% wine, or 42.53 g (1.5 oz.) of 40% liquor.[37]

An insult to women is the "weed tampon", promoted as a THC-infused suppository for the relief of menstrual cramps. The advertisements on the web for these products make claims that the products include THC, CBD and organic cocoa butter. One producer claims that their "weed" is grown outdoors in Northern California without the use of pesticides.[38]

THE INSULT TO SCIENCE   The indisputable evidence of harm associated with tobacco products was available for decades before the public came to accept it, adjust their tolerance, and subsequently the use of these dangerous products. The tobacco industry used tactics of delay and denial to buy the time needed to find replacement smokers and new markets. It is well known that they targeted both female and youth. By denying the evidence that now exists that establishes marijuana harms, the emerging marijuana industry has bought time to expand. Delay, deny and distract, all strategies and the track record of Big Tobacco.

"People have been consuming cannabis around the world for the last 5000 years and there's no known reports of cannabis causing illness or causing death."[39] —Brendan Kennedy. Professor Leslie Walker, with Adolescent Medicine at the Seattle Children's Hospital, in a follow up to the remark made by Brendan Kennedys on *Cannabis Inc.*, reported: "Absolutely there's evidence that marijuana causes illness—in real life, in daily life, in research there's volumes of evidence that it causes illness."[39]

"Yeah, it's a psycho active substance but compared to alcohol it's nothing. I mean as far as the impact to health, as far as the impact to society. I mean it's really a fairly benign substance," said John Davis, marijuana activist.[40]

"What is already known is that in casual users, THC can disrupt focus, working memory, decision making and motivation for 24 hours. The fact that we can see these structural effects in the brain could indicate that the effects of THC are longer lasting than we previously thought," said Dr. Jodi Gilman.[41]

Should you worry about marijuana edibles in your kid's Halloween treats? Law Enforcement is warning parents about the dangers of cannabis-infused sweets. But it might just be a lot of huffing and puffing: Headline; October 30, 2014, *TheGuardian.com.* "There are no long-lasting negative impacts (underlined) from consuming cannabis, and most of any discomfort fades away following, a long, deep sleep."- "Is marijuana deadly? Absolutely not, as proven by science....If young people do manage to get into a marijuana stash, intentionally or accidently, parents should remember that cannabis is one of the safest substances known to man, with no toxicity and no long term effects (underlined)."[42] —Jodie Emery— also referred to as the "Princess of Pot". This was not a quote out of Grimm's Fairy Tales.

The NORML of North Carolina official blog states that the plant really is a medicine and that it really is safe.[43]

Frequent or long term marijuana use may significantly increase a man's risk of developing the most aggressive type of testicular cancer.[44] This form of cancer tends to strike young men, between the ages of 20 and 25, and accounts for about 40% of all testicular cancer cases.[44]

"Epidemiological evidence in the public domain not only identifies cannabis use as a risk factor for schizophrenia, but in individuals with a predisposition for schizophrenia, it results in an exacerbation of symptoms and worsening of the schizophrenic prognosis."[45] —Kathy Gyngell (UK)

Dr. Chris Colwell, Chief of Emergency Medicine at the Denver Health Center, told *CBS4 News* out of Denver, Colorado that five to ten times each week people enter the Denver Health emergency department after ingesting marijuana and acting suicidal who need to be restrained so as to not be a danger to themselves other people.[46]

"Cannabis is far stronger these days and we are seeing the emergence of a new severe form of emphysema—which could lead to people struggling for breath for the rest of their life. We urgently need a detailed study across the UK which analyses the national picture of cannabis-use and lung disease," said Dr. Damian Mckeon.[47]

In December 2014, the UK media reported that the country needed to be prepared for a steep rise in the number of young adults affected by a severe form of lung disease, due to their regular cannabis and tobacco use.[48] Severe emphysema was beginning to show up, affecting young to middle aged people who used illicit drugs. It was further reported that researchers were warning that lungs may become damaged more quickly in cannabis users, who smoke the drug with tobacco.

"Even in the seven participants who smoked only once a week, there was evidence of structural differences in two significant regions of the brain. The more the subjects smoked, the greater the differences."[49] —Dr. (Hans) Breiter. Dr. Breiter reported seeing changes in the nucleus accumbens among adults in their early 20s, who had smoked daily for three years but who had stopped for at least two years.[49]

"In February of 2017, University of California Davis Medical Center doctors published an article in Clinical Microbiology and Infection. They reported that some of their cancer patients undergoing intensive chemotherapy had acquired fungal infections in their lungs. The doctors teamed up with a drug testing laboratory, gathered samples from medical marijuana dispensaries across California, and tested them thoroughly. They were shocked by the test results: 90 percent of the samples were contaminated with bacteria, other pathogens, and fungi, including a type like the one that infected their patients, who it turned out were using marijuana to allay their chemotherapy-induced nausea. The patients were young and had beatable cancers. But one died, not from his cancer but from his fungal infection. Doctors warn that patients with compromised immune systems should not smoke marijuana, which provides the avenue for fungi to enter the lungs and cause infection....CNN's Sanjay Gupta, MD, gave the commercial marijuana industry a huge boost when he produced three documentaries called Weed (2014), declaring 'science is clearly' on the side of pot."[50] —National Families in Action

"We have seen an increase in unintentional ingestion of

marijuana by children since the modification of drug laws in Colorado," said George Wang, M.D., clinical instructor in pediatrics at Children's Hospital in Colorado at the University of Colorado – School of Medicine.[51] Dr. Wang and Michael Kosnett, M.D., M.P.H., testified before a state advisory panel to recommend they bring in child resistant packaging for marijuana edibles. Governor Hickenlooper called upon the Colorado Department of Revenue's new Marijuana Enforcement Division to create requirements similar to the federal Poison Prevention Packaging Act of 1970.[52]

"The courts may serve as another avenue of regulation. Consumers who are injured by ingestion of edibles may bring personal-injury claims seeking damages against manufacturers and retailers. Judges and juries could well find credible consumers' claims that these products were negligently designed, since the risks of overdose and consumption by children are reasonably foreseeable and avoidable. Such lawsuits could make the effects of these products on health more salient for manufacturers—but might be too infrequent and low-cost to spur adoption of more responsible business practices. Lawsuits would be more likely to draw attention to the problem than to obviate the need for formal regulations."[53] —Robert MacCoun, Professor Faculty of Law, Stanford University

18. Creative Means

A Colorado pot shop closed after a Washington-based group, opposed to legal marijuana, sued not just the pot shop but a list of firms doing business with it, including the landlord and accountant.[1]

"With another lawsuit pending in southern Colorado, the cases represent a new approach to fighting marijuana."[2] —"It is still illegal to cultivate, sell or possess marijuana under federal law," said Brian Barnes, lawyer for Safe Streets Alliance, a Washington-based anti-crime group that brought the lawsuits on behalf of neighbors of the two Colorado pot businesses."[2] "If our legal theory works, basically what it will mean is that folks who are participating in the marijuana industry in any capacity are exposing themselves to pretty significant liability," said Barnes. *Racketeering Law Suits Target Colorado Marijuana Industry*, Kristen Wyatt, *Associated Press*, July 13, 2015.[3]

The 1970, *Racketeer Influenced and Corrupt Organizations Act (RICO)*, sets up federal criminal penalties for activity that benefits a criminal enterprise. *RICO* also provides for civil lawsuits, by people hurt by such racketeering. In the case coming forward in Colorado the neighbors, of the two businesses, allege the pot businesses could hurt their property values. Lawsuits, initiating from the governments of Nebraska and Oklahoma, allege violations of the RICO statutes.[4] In these cases the alleged offenses are violations of federal law, including the manufacturing and distribution of marijuana, conspiracy, money laundering, maintaining drug properties, investing in drug operations, using communications to facilitate drug trafficking and many others. The defendants in the case include the Governor of Colorado and the Executive Director of the Colorado Department of Revenue and others. All of the defendants are charged with facilitating and promoting the marijuana industry through licensing, taxing and regulation of entities that are violating a number of federal laws.[4]

G. Robert Blakey, professor of law at Notre Dame Law School in Indiana, and a former United States federal prosecutor, authored the *U.S. Racketeer Influenced and Corrupt Organizations Act*. The *RICO* statute was passed to facilitate prosecution of members of organized crime. Professor Blakey has compared the structure of the tobacco industry with the Mafia and recommended criminal prosecution of tobacco companies and their executives: "This is the organization of the tobacco industry. Now, what do they do over here? A pattern of racketeering activity. Let me show you that pattern. This is the industry's scheme to defraud. Here's the statute again. Person, enterprise, pattern of racketeering activity. And here it is, the intentional sale of a defective product that's both addictive and lethal. The failure to market a safer product. And you can go down this list at each stage, taken collectively, these are the trees of the forest to show that this product was no longer legitimate and legitimately marketed.

It's illegitimate and illegitimately marketed. And in

particular, targeted to the children. Despite the fact that in fifty states the sale of cigarettes to children is illegal. This is not a legal product when it's sold to children. It's the same thing functionally as cocaine or heroin. This is a drug industry. Not a tobacco industry. *RICO* was designed to deal with the (illegal) drug industry. And that's exactly what it does in this situation. It's just that the drug, instead of heroin and cocaine, is nicotine."[5]   Frontline TV

Another legal claim involves a Holiday Inn in Colorado.[6] A marijuana manufacturing and retail sales business is being built across the street from the hotel. The hotel alleges it is losing business.

The Marijuana Policy Project's director of communications Mason Tvert sent out a public response encouraging the individuals who support legalizing marijuana to join their nationwide boycott of Holiday Inn hotels until the suit was withdrawn, and also to sign their petition urging the hotel operator to withdraw their legal suit.[7] He further claimed that the people behind the effort were former warriors in the Ronald Reagan administration. He also asked for help in sending businesses a message that they would face consequences if they joined the fight to keep the prohibition of marijuana in place.[7]

It was reported that U.S. Hershey CO. settled a trademark infringement lawsuits against marijuana companies in Colorado and Washington State, both of whom the candy maker said had sold products in packaging that resembled its wrappers.[8]

In 2014 an ad campaign, aimed at discouraging teen marijuana use, was unveiling in Denver, Colorado. The campaign featured 9' tall human-sized rat cages with signage that read; "Don't Be a Lab Rat. Because so much is still unknown about pot's effects on kids brains, teens who do smoke it become unwitting research subjects."[9] Television ads were part of the $2 million dollar campaign that offered the warning: "If you're younger than 25, smoking marijuana means you're gambling on losing IQ points."[9] The marijuana lobby criticized the campaign and called it "fear-mongering".[10]

THE ERRONEOUS NOTION OF INEVITABILITY California in 2010 rejected the ballot initiative *Proposition 19* that would have legalize marijuana; the state represents 12% of the American eligible voters. In 2014, 345 cities in California had bans or moratoriums against marijuana dispensaries who sell marijuana for medical purposes, 46 cities had limited dispensaries to industrial zones, with no commercial or residential areas permitted. The data is from 2014, as reported by the Coalition for a Drug Free California.[11]

The City of San Jose, being the third largest city in the State of California, and the tenth largest in the United States, was anticipated to be a big win for the Pro-Marijuana Advocates. The city has banned marijuana dispensaries in their community through a civic ordinance.[11] All attempts by the pro-marijuana advocates to attack these cities in the courts to override their bans have failed; all the way to the California Supreme Court. The California Supreme Court ruled unanimously that cities and counties have the right to ban medical marijuana dispensaries within their borders, despite the existence of a state law. The court ruled that the scope of the *Compassionate Use Act of 1996* and other related state law is "limited and circumscribed".[12]

In July of 2015, the Arizona Republican Party released the results of a poll that showed 58% of likely voters would vote in opposition to the legalization of marijuana, with only 31% supporting the measure and only 11% undecided.[13] Arizona defeated the ballot initiative to legalize non-medical use in 2016.

The election cycle of 2016 did see successful ballot initiatives for the marijuana interests but it also saw defeats. The path to full national legalization is far from an inevitable conclusion, as more and more interest groups respond to the experiments on legalization currently underway.

As of 2015, accounting for 321 total local jurisdictions in Colorado, 71% prohibited any medical or recreational marijuana businesses, 21% allowed any medical and recreational marijuana businesses, with 8% allowing either medical or recreational marijuana businesses, not both.[14] In August of 2015, poll results out of Colorado showed that the popularity for marijuana legalization was lagging. The measure was losing support over concerns of traffic problems, youth usage, child exposures and the proliferation of edible marijuana products.[14]

19. Promoting to Voters

The Alaska voters successfully warded off the marijuana lobby by rejecting a ballot initiative to legalize marijuana in 2010. Medi-pot had previously been voted into law in Alaska in 1998. The pot lobby went once again after marijuana for non-medical use in Alaska in 2014, and they won.

The pro-legalization campaign used the slogan —*Impact on the Consumer* and issued a statement in an effort to sway voters to their side.[1] The information in a con and rebuttal format was also posted on the public website of Ballotpedia: "Many people die from alcohol use. Nobody dies from marijuana use. People die from alcohol overdoses. There has never been a fatal marijuana overdose. The health-related costs associated with alcohol use far exceed those of marijuana use. Alcohol use damages the brain. Marijuana use does not. (Despite the myths we've heard throughout our lives about marijuana killing brain cells, it turns out that a growing number of studies seem to indicate that marijuana actually has neuroprotective properties. This means that it works to protect brain cells from harm.)

Alcohol use is linked to cancer. Marijuana use is not. Surprisingly, the researchers found that people who smoked marijuana actually had lower incidences of cancer compared to non-users of the drug. Alcohol is more addictive than marijuana whereas marijuana has not been found to produce any symptoms of physical withdrawal.

Alcohol use increases the risk of injury to the consumer. Marijuana does not. Alcohol use contributes to aggressive and violent behavior. Marijuana use does not. Alcohol use is a major factor in violent crimes. Marijuana use is not. Alcohol use contributes to the likelihood of domestic abuse and sexual assault. Marijuana use does not."[2]

In October 2015, The Marijuana Control Board of Alaska, released a 100-page report—*Labelling of all marijuana products would be required to state the following warnings*: "Marijuana has intoxicating effects and may be habit forming. Marijuana can impair concentration, coordination, and judgement. Do not operate a vehicle or machinery under its influence. There may be health risks associated with consumption of marijuana. For use only by adults twenty-one and older. Keep out of reach of children. Marijuana should not be used by women who are pregnant or breast feeding."[3] The long, slow, difficult job of correcting erroneous statements lies ahead for the officials running public health in the fine state of Alaska.

The Alaska 2014 pro-on legalize campaign contributors included; The Marijuana Policy Project, The Drug Policy Alliance. The opposition, under the banner *Big Marijuana Big Mistake Vote No on 2*, included support from Anchorage Municipal Assembly, Alaska Association of Police Chiefs, Napaskiak Tribal Council, Bristol Bay Native Corporation, Chenega Corporation, Alaska Conference of Mayors, and Alaska Regional Hospital. The Marijuana Policy Project invested over $1.1 million in Alaska versus the $189,000 that was raised in opposition.[4]

Alaska Marijuana Legalization, *Ballot Measure 2* (2014) was approved, which allows people age 21 and older to possess up to one ounce of marijuana and up to six plants.

In Florida the *United for Care* was heavily financed by lawyer, John Morgan. Proponents raised close to $8.1 million to legalize marijuana for medical purposes in 2014.[5] Florida was the first of 23 states where opponents were able to raise significant funds. *No on 2* raised $6.4 million.[6] *United for Care* was defeated in the November election.

PUSH POLLS The practice of "push polling" has been employed to influence voters and legislators into thinking that the majority supports legalization. The practice of "push polling" and the skewing of polling questions, could be and should be minimized by requiring that the exact wording of the questions posed be included with results commentary released through the media.

Polling commissioned by the Government of Canada in 2013, on public opinion regarding cannabis control, showed 31% of women and 40% of men thought marijuana should be legalized and taxed.[5] 34% of women and 33% of men said it should be decriminalized for small amounts.[7]

The results of the polling were reported in the Canadian media.[8] The Canadian Centre on Addiction and Mental Health writing on the poll had this to say: "Public opinion on cannabis control has shifted considerably in the past decade. Ten years ago about half of Canadians believed cannabis use should be decriminalized or legalized; today, about two thirds of Canadians hold that view."[6] The question asked: How Do Canadians Feel about Marijuana? It should be legalized and taxed—

response women 31% men 40%? It should be decriminalized for small amounts. Response women 34% men 33%.[8]
Add the number of men and women together you get roughly
two-thirds—if you add the response to legalization and
decriminalization together you get similar results. What is
missing is the word "either".

The IPSOS REID polling of 2014 showed the Canadian
support for legalization had risen to 37%.[9] In 2015, support
rose with the increasing interest in Justin Trudeau as leader
of the Liberal Party of Canada and candidate for Prime
Minister. Trudeau had announced his intentions to legalize marijuana in 2012 and campaigned on the issue in 2015.
IPSOS REID found that by 2015, 65% of Canadians were in
favor of decriminalization.[10]

"It is difficult to judge whether shift in public opinion represents the "celebrity effect", uncertainty of the meaning of
the terms, a progressive movement away from laws considered
oppressive, or normalization of cannabis use as a large majority
in that poll did not consider marijuana laws to be a high priority matter."[11] —Harold Kalant, M.D., Ph.D. Toronto, Canada

On August 8, 2015, The *Vancouver Province* reported on
polling conducted, after the *Maclean's Magazine* leadership
debate, by Mainstreet Research: "Trudeau, however, won the
debate, if only slightly. Twenty-six per cent of respondents
thought the Liberal leader won, followed by Mulcair (23),
May (22) and Harper (20)," said Quito Maggi, President of
Mainstreet Research Polling.[12]

On February 20, 2014, Jeff Jedras, as a "special" to the
National Post interviewed Quito Maggi: "We have two goals,"
said Quito Maggi, a veteran political organizer serving as

campaign director for Legalize Canada. "Work in the next election to elect Members of Parliament who support legalization in all 338 ridings, and keep pressure on Parliament after the election to make good on their promises and implement cannabis law reform."[13] The article continues: "Legalize Canada is pan-partisan, said Maggi, a prominent Liberal organizer." [13] The title of the article for the story: *Liberals Get Help From Pro-Pot Group. A new lobby group has a $7 million budget and a two-year plan to elect Members of Parliament who support the legalization of marijuana.*[14]

Gallup poll results released on November 6, 2014, showed that the support for the legalization of marijuana was falling in the United States.[16] The poll also showed that the support for legalization at 64% for democrats and at 39% for republicans.[16] Age 18-29: 60% in favor of legalization; Age 30-44: 57% in favor of legalization; Age 45-64: 41% in favor of legalization; Age 65 and older: 37% in favor of legalization.[16]

The Gallup question asked Americans: "*Do you think the use of marijuana should be made legal, or not?*

2014 —yes 51%, no 47%, no opinion 2% and in 2013 —yes 58%, no 39%, no opinion 3%.[16] —Gallup

The drop in popular support for the legalization of marijuana in United States by 7% in 2014 is worth reviewing. Since 1969 only three Gallup poll results have showed a majority of people affirming legalization, for all remaining years the majority expressed their opposition. The drop of 7% in 2014 may well reflect a "softness" in the electorate on the issue. Given the majority of the electorate do not use marijuana products, mild agitation could further erode support for legalization. The electorate does not need to be called to frenetic action, just agitated to the point of saying, or voting "no" when asked for their views.

Over one hundred cities and town, roughly one-third of the communities in Massachusetts have now banned or restricted marijuana businesses since voters legalized the drug for non-medical use in 2016. The reality has set in for the many residents who do not use marijuana. "Asking people whether marijuana should be legal is hardly the same as asking if they want pot shops in their neighborhoods."[17] —Geoffrey Beckwith, executive director of the Massachusetts Municipal Association.

The vast majority of the electorate in both Canada and the USA do not use marijuana, and for those that have ever-used the majority have rejected it as an ongoing, viable lifestyle choice.

MARKETING MARIJUANA PRODUCTS "A majority of parents identify the number one place where it should be permissible to advertise marijuana as "nowhere."[18] —*ZERO Drug Free Marijuana Survey.*

"(Canadian) *Bill-C-45* prohibits any promotion, packaging and labelling of cannabis that could be appealing to young persons or encourages its consumption, while allowing consumers to have access to information with which they can make informed decisions...It also bans the displaying of marijuana products in retail outlets where they can be seen by young persons and prohibits any marijuana marketing that depicts a person, character or animal or any association with a glamorous or relaxed lifestyle."[19] —*Bill C.45* The proposed law does not call for plain packaging as had been recommended by the task force.

Several licensed marijuana producers in March of 2017 sent a letter to the Prime Minister and the federal cabinet in which they argued that a lack of brand awareness and advertising would thwart their efforts to differentiate themselves from the black market.

"The legislation seemed to leave the door open to alcohol rather than tobacco-level advertising restrictions, said Brendan Kennedy, president of Tilray, one of the licensed producers behind the letter.[20] "It seems like a positive step and it seems like it's not going the way of plain packaging, which I think would be a huge disservice to consumers. Brand prohibition would create a race to the bottom where essentially companies would compete on price and potency, which is the exact opposite of what the government wants," concluded Kennedy in an interview.[20]

In December of 2014, The Harbor House of Dank in San Pedro, California hired an artist to paint both Santa smoking a joint and a snowman holding a prescription pill bottle. Hundreds of outraged people forced the owner to take down the pot-smoking Santa. The 24 hour marijuana store spread the images across social media.[21]

"A powerful marijuana industry lobby has emerged that sued Colorado to stop restrictions on advertising to protect children, and is now pushing back against municipal regulations to keep pot stores away from schools and day care facilities in other states," said Kevin Sabet, Ph.D. [22]

"All kids were told smoking was bad—and was only for adults—who created, in part, its impressive appeal. And this appeal was anything but natural. It was the studied and meticulous invention of the industry (tobacco) that would come to understand—and exploit-critical aspects of motivation, psychology, and human biology."[23] —Allen M. Brandt, *The Cigarette Century*

For all the benefit of early and continued drug education, children and youth remain exposed to the powerful messaging, marketing tactics, and reach of Big Marijuana. Youth are weaned off protective messaging, seduced into the world of drugs.

Warning signs that your child or teenager maybe involved in drugs: A sudden change in school grades could signal something else other than academic performance has become a priority; sudden changes in attitudes, including lethargy, hyperactivity, anger or violent outbursts, newly displayed aggression, a sudden and significant change in weight, a decline in personal hygiene, and medical signs such as tremors, slurred speech, or other symptoms that are out of the ordinary.[24]

20. The Tobacco Template

California GFarmaLab, with the use of automation, has developed the capability of producing 8,000 pre-rolled marijuana cigarettes a day, or filling 100 vape cartridges in 30 seconds.[1]

In 1913, R.J. Reynolds pushed out a nationally coordinated advertising campaign and product launch for rolled and packaged Camel cigarettes. The same full-page ad appeared in dozens of newspapers across America, marking the first time a consumer product had been marketed in such an extensive way. In one year, 425 million packages of Camel cigarettes were sold and the success of the Reynolds' campaign made marketing history.[2]

Cigarette and smokeless tobacco companies spend billions of dollars annually to market their products. In 2014, the industry spent more than $9 billion on advertising and promotional expenses in the United States alone; paid out as price discounts to retailers and wholesalers, payments for stocking, displaying particular brands and for volume rebates, and other promotions.[3]

Matthew L. Myers, President of the Campaign for Tobacco-Free Kids, on January 10, 2017 responded to the first comprehensive review of the economic impact of tobacco use and global tobacco control efforts in nearly 20 years, *The Economics of Tobacco and Tobacco Control*: "The tobacco industry's deep pockets and deadly tactics remain the greatest obstacle to progress in addressing the devastating global toll of tobacco use. The report notes that in addition to continued implementation of evidence-based tobacco control strategies, vigilant monitoring of the tobacco industry's ongoing efforts to promote tobacco use and undermine tobacco control is crucial."[4]

Tobacco product advertising and promotions influence young people to take up the use of tobacco products, as evidenced by the fact that the three most advertised brands are the preferred brands of cigarettes smoked by adolescents and young adults.[5]

"The tobacco industry's message is unmistakeable. There is no need to worry because the more than 20 terminal tobacco diseases that constitute the tobacco epidemic are brought to you by a "legal", normal industry selling a "legal", normal product."[6] —Garfield Mahood, (former) Executive Director (1976-2011), Non-Smoker's Rights Association of Canada.

The legalization of tobacco products and the condoning of their promotion has proven to be the most grievous mistake, in terms of health outcomes, the world has ever known. For over six decades public health advocates have been fighting back the advances of the tobacco industry and it has proven to be a tremendously costly and difficult battle. The devastation caused by the sale of tobacco products continues to this day, as the industry continues to prosper.

"The 2013 profits of the top six tobacco companies are equivalent to the combined profits of The Coca-Cola Company, Walt Disney, General Mills, FedEx, AT&T, Google,

McDonald's and Starbucks in the same year."[7] —Tobacco Atlas

In spite of heavy taxes and advertising restrictions, selling cigarettes and other tobacco products in the U.S. continues to be highly profitable. Altria recorded approximately $24 billion in sales and $4.3 billion in profits in 2013.[8]

Globally, tobacco use is increasingly concentrated among the poor and other vulnerable groups and accounts for a significant share of health disparities between the wealthy and those living in poverty. The August 2012 results, of the largest-ever study on global tobacco use, *The Global Adult Tobacco Study*, showed that an estimated 49% of men and 11% of women, in developing countries, smoked and or had used smokeless tobacco.[9]

An estimated 5.8 trillion cigarettes were smoked worldwide in 2014, and consumption continues to rise.[10] As the African population is growing more rapidly than other regions of the world it is anticipated, that in the absence of comprehensive smoking prevention protocols, the region's smoking prevalence rate will continue to climb over the next decade. The result of this growth in tobacco product consumption will be tremendous devastation, in terms of health outcomes and socioeconomic damage, to African families.

"Tobacco killed one hundred million people worldwide in the 20th. century—and if current trends continue, it will kill one billion people in the 21st century. Every year, tobacco kills more than 480,000 Americans and six million people worldwide. The vast majority started smoking as children."[11] —Campaign for Tobacco-Free Kids

Many adolescents who smoke are nicotine dependent. *The Youth Risk Behavior Survey*, a 2007 survey of students in grades 9–12 in the United States, found that 60.9% of students who ever smoked cigarettes daily tried to quit, with only 12.2% becoming smoke-free.[12]

Many opportunities to effectively curtail Big Tobacco have been lost over the years, and this harsh reality should guide the electorate and policy makers as they deliberate over the legalization and commercialization of the marijuana industry. Given the history of tobacco's corporate behavior, it is seriously questioned whether regulatory agencies will effectively limit the promotion of "legal" m-cigarettes and adequately patrol the activities of Big Marijuana.

"This industry is not about hippies singing *Kumbaya* in a drum circle and smoking a few joints. It's about businessmen in suits making billions. They see bags of money for them and they're going after it like any other industry would."[13]
—Kevin Sabet, Ph.D.

As marijuana commercialization remains illegal under US federal law the major American stock exchanges have not accepted listings from marijuana businesses, and institutional bankers and lenders have stayed away from these this sector.

A *Bloomberg News* story, *Cannabis Two-Step: Raise Cash in Canada, Spend It in U.S.*, written by Jack Kaskey, appeared in the spring of 2017.[14]The journalist explains how an investment banker, formerly with Goldman Sachs Group Inc., left the USA and came to Canada and proceeded to raise significant funds in Canada through the creation of a public company. The funds were then used for marijuana business activities back in the USA. The company was listed on the Canadian Stock Exchange and began trading in September of 2016, raising more than $50 million Canadian through a public offering underwritten by Canada's largest nonbank brokerage firm.

It was reported by Kaskey, that the monies raised had been used to invest in marijuana operations, including in marijuana retail dispensaries in Colorado, Massachusetts, Vermont and New Mexico.[14]

"There appears to be a current blindness to corporate agenda/greed and conflict of interest. The primary benefactors of the legalization process will be corporate interests and those who pay will be the disempowered—a group that is growing exponentially." —Ray Baker, M.D., F.C.F.P., F.A.S.A.M.

Tobacco industry once had high hopes for marijuana business, appeared in the *Los Angeles Times* in June of 2014, in which journalist Evan Halper elaborated on information revealed in internal tobacco industry documents, which had been discussed in the Milbank Quarterly earlier in the same week.[15]

Tobacco documents show as the American populace moved to greater use and acceptance of marijuana in the 1960s and 1970s, with talk of legalization, the tobacco industry had identified the possibility of their entry into the marijuana market.[15] Halper reports how in 1969 a vice-president at Philip Morris corresponded with the USA Justice Department's narcotic bureau, for the purpose of obtaining marijuana for the tobacco company's research on a potential product.[15] A special permit to grow, cultivate and make marijuana extracts was reportedly issued.[15,16]

In a report commissioned by the cigarette manufacturer Brown and Williamson, industry representatives discuss the company's capabilities in terms of creating an alternative product line.[17]

"The tobacco companies may deny even thinking about it, but they have to think about it," said Gerry Sullivan, portfolio manager of the Vice Fund, a $300 million mutual fund made up of alcohol, tobacco, gambling and defense company stocks.[18] "It is an opportunity to diversify their business and help benefit shareholders," Sullivan said. "That is what management is most likely pursuing in the dark corners of some research lab in Virginia."[15] —Evan Halper, *Los Angeles Times*

"Addiction is big business, and with legal marijuana it's only getting bigger. Not surprisingly, Big Tobacco is also getting on the marijuana bandwagon. Manufacturers Altria and Brown & Williamson have registered domain names that include the words "marijuana" and "cannabis." Imagine how much they will spend peddling their new brand of addiction to our kids. We cannot sit by while these companies open a new front in their battle against our children's health."[17a] —Patrick J. Kennedy

"ALTRIAMARIJUANA.COM" —"ALTRIACANNABIS.COM" Altria is the parent company of Phillip Morris, the manufacturer of *Marlboro, Players, Benson & Hedges*, along with other popular brands of tobacco cigarettes. "Altria has significant potential in the marijuana industry, if legalization occurs Altria and other large tobacco corporations will have strong competitive advantages over smaller businesses in distribution, marketing, brand strength and economies of scale. If Altria can capitalize on the marijuana market as well as it has on cigarettes, the company will nearly double in size."[19] —Ben Reynolds, *The Street* (MSN)

Tobacco companies have been interested in marijuana and marijuana legalization as both a potential and a rival product since at least the 1970s relayed researchers Rachel Ann Barry, Heikki Hiilamo and Stanton A. Glantz, in a June 2014 paper for the *Milbank Quarterly*.[20]

"As public opinion shifted and governments began relaxing laws pertaining to marijuana criminalization, the tobacco companies modified their corporate planning strategies to prepare for future consumer demand....Legalizing marijuana opens the market to major corporations, including tobacco companies, which have the financial resources, product design technology to optimize puff-by-puff delivery of a psychoactive drug (nicotine), marketing muscle, and political clout to transform the marijuana market." [21] —*Waiting for the Opportune Moment: The Tobacco Industry and Marijuana Legalization.*

"Legal pot is set to outsell the breakfast of champions,"[20] *Bloomberg* reporter, Shelly Banjo tweeted. In 2019, US sales of legal marijuana are predicted to reach $11.6 billion, surpassing ready-to-eat breakfast cereal sales, by more than $2 billion.[22]

Researchers from the ArcView Group, a cannabis industry investment and research firm based in California, claims that the U.S. market for legal cannabis grew 74% in 2014 to $2.7 billion, up from $1.3 billion in 2013.[23] The research firm found legal cannabis sales jumped 17% to $5.4 billion in 2015, and projected sales in the US would reach 6.7 billion in the next year, which was shy of the $6.9 billion actually reached in terms of sales for 2016.[24] Sales are projected to increase to $21.6 billion by 2021, with a 26% compound annual growth rate.[25]

PROFITEERING Journalist Susan Adams of *Forbes Trep Talks* in 2016 asked Jake Heimark, a principal of Plus Gum —a Palo Alto-based company that makes cannabis-infused chewing gum, why he had chosen to start a marijuana company.[26] "A friend sent me the *60 Minutes* piece on cannabis and said: 'Look at this market. It's completely new and undefined. I knew nothing about cannabis....We think there will be an influx of capital from the tobacco and liquor industry and maybe the food industry. Our goal is to become as large as possible, with as much brand presence as possible. We want either to be too large to be competed with or the entry play for one of those companies."[26]

LESSONS FROM AN IDENTIFIED KILLER There is no safe level of exposure to second-hand tobacco smoke. In 2004, children accounted for 28% of the deaths attributable to second-hand smoke, and every year more than 42,000 Americans die second-hand smoke deaths, including 900 infants.[27,28]

In the United States, more than $156 billion a year of productivity is lost due to deaths from tobacco and diseases caused by second-hand smoke, with $170 billion going to direct medical costs for smokers yearly.[29] Only 18% of the world's population, are protected by comprehensive national smoke-free laws.[26] Breathing second-hand marijuana smoke could damage heart and blood vessels as much as second-hand cigarette smoke, according to preliminary research presented at the American Heart Association's Scientific Sessions in 2014.[30] "Most people know second-hand cigarette smoke is bad for you, but many don't realize that second-hand marijuana smoke may also be harmful," said Matthew Springer, Ph.D., cardiovascular researcher and associate professor of Medicine at the University of California, San Francisco's Cardiology Division.[31]

Second-hand exposure to cannabis smoke under "*extreme conditions*", such as an unventilated room or enclosed vehicle, can cause non-smokers to feel the effects of the drug, have minor problems with memory and coordination, and in some cases test positive for the drug in a urinalysis.[32] Those are the findings of a Johns Hopkins University School of Medicine study, reported in the Journal Drug and Alcohol Dependence in 2015.[32] "We found positive drug effects in the first few hours, a mild sense of intoxication and mild impairment on measures of cognitive performance," said senior author Ryan Vandrey, Ph.D., an associate professor of psychiatry and behavioral sciences at Johns Hopkins University.[29] He added; "These were relatively slight effects, but even so, some participants did not pass the equivalent of a workplace drug test."

In September 2009, marijuana smoke was added to the list of "chemicals" known to the state of California to cause cancer or reproductive toxicity by the California Environmental Protection Agency Office of Environmental Health Hazards.[33]

The decision to add marijuana smoke to the list was reached in consideration of the August 2009 report; *Evidence on the Carcinogenicity of Marijuana Smoke,* which had been prepared by The Office of Environmental Health Hazard Assessment's (OEHHA) Reproductive and Cancer Hazard Assessment Branch. The report concludes: "There is evidence from some epidemiological studies of marijuana smoke suggestive of increased cancer risk from both direct and parental marijuana smoking. However, this evidence is limited by validity issues and small numbers of studies for most types of cancer. Direct marijuana smoking has been statistically significantly associated with cancer of the lung, head and neck, bladder, brain, and testis. Parental marijuana smoking before or during gestation has been statistically significantly associated with childhood cancer. Childhood cancers that have been associated with **maternal** marijuana smoking are acute myeloid leukemia, neuroblastoma, and rhabdomyosarcoma. Childhood cancers that have been associated with **paternal** marijuana smoking are leukemia (all types), infant leukemia (all types), acute lymphoblastic leukemia, acute myeloid leukemia, and rhabdomyosarcoma....

There is evidence that marijuana smoke is genotoxic, immunosuppressive, and can alter endocrine function.

Studies of Δ9-THC and other cannabinoids provide evidence for alterations of multiple cell signaling pathways, in endocrine function, and suppression of the innate and adaptive immune response. Prolonged exposures to marijuana smoke in animals and humans cause proliferative and inflammatory lesions in the lung. Marijuana smoke and tobacco smoke share many characteristics with regard to chemical composition and toxicological activity. Tobacco smoke is a *Proposition 65* carcinogen, and at least 33 individual constituents present in both marijuana smoke and tobacco smoke are *Proposition 65* carcinogens."

The preface to the report provided a background to the formation of both the report and the conclusions that were reached: *The Safe Drinking Water and Toxic Enforcement Act* of 1986 (*Proposition 65, California Health and Safety Code 25249.5 et seq.*) requires that the Governor cause to be published a list of those chemicals "known to the state" to cause cancer or reproductive toxicity.

The Act specifies that "a chemical is known to the state to cause cancer or reproductive toxicity—if in the opinion of the state's qualified experts the chemical has been clearly shown through scientifically valid testing according to generally accepted principles to cause cancer or reproductive toxicity The lead agency for implementing *Proposition 65* is the Office of Environmental Health Hazard Assessment (OEHHA) of the California Environmental Protection Agency. The "state's qualified experts" regarding findings of carcinogenicity are identified as the members of the Carcinogen Identification Committee (CIC) of the OEHHA Science Advisory Board.

OEHHA announced the selection of marijuana smoke as a chemical for consideration for listing by the CIC in the California Regulatory Notice Register on December 12, 2007, subsequent to consultation with the Committee at their November 19, 2007 meeting. At that meeting, the Committee advised OEHHA to prepare hazard identification materials for marijuana smoke.

The December 12th notice also marked the start of a 60-day public request for information relevant to the assessment of the evidence on the carcinogenicity marijuana smoke. No information was received as a result of this request. This document was released as a draft document in March 2009 for a 60-day public comment period. No public comments were received. The draft document provided the Committee with the available scientific evidence on the carcinogenic potential of this chemical. The current document was the final version of the document that was discussed by the Committee at their May 29, 2009 meeting. At their May 29, 2009 meeting the Committee, by a vote of five in favor and one against, found that marijuana smoke had been 'clearly shown through scientifically valid testing according to generally accepted principles to cause cancer.' Accordingly, marijuana smoke was placed on the *Proposition 65* list of chemicals known to the state to cause cancer."[34]

The *Monitoring Health Concerns Related to Marijuana in Colorado 2016* report estimated that for Colorado in 2015, sixteen thousand children between the ages of one and four-teen, were possibly exposed to second-hand marijuana smoke or vapor in their homes. Although this is only an estimation, and a possible outcome, it is a concern worthy of mention, as well as further investigation.[35]

A study released in 2016 found that one in six infants and toddlers, admitted to a Colorado hospital with coughing, wheezing and exhibiting other symptoms of bronchiolitis, also tested positive for marijuana exposure.[33] The study, *Marijuana Exposure in Children Hospitalized for Bronchiolitis,* recruited parents of previously healthy children, between one month of age and two years old, who were admitted to Children's Hospital Colorado (CHC) between January 2013 and April 2014, with bronchiolitis.[33] Urine samples showed traces of a metabolite of tetrahydrocannabinol (THC), the psychoactive component of marijuana, in 16% of the children. It was further discovered that 21% of children were THC positive after legal-ization in 2012, compared with 10% before.[36]

"The findings suggest that second-hand marijuana smoke, which contains carcinogenic and psychoactive chemicals, may be a rising child health concern as marijuana increas-ingly becomes legal for medical and recreational use in the United States," said lead researcher, Karen M. Wilson, M.D, M.P.H, F.A.A.P., an associate professor of pediatrics at the University of Colorado School of Medicine, and section head at Children's Hospital Colorado.[37] The study concluded that marijuana should never be smoked around children.

A SMOKE-FREE HOME Canadian family courts have ordered that children under the care of a primary care of a guardian or a parent are to be protected from second-hand tobacco cigarette smoke exposure and to order that there shall be no smoking within a child's home or within the family vehicle.

21. E-cigarettes Pave the Way

The arrival of e-cigarettes in 2006, offered a smoke-free delivery device and a partial solution to the problem that second hand smoking laws had placed with the tobacco industry; which was the marginalization of smokers, by those that had come to abhor smoking and feared exposure to second and third-hand smoke.

Tobacco firms welcomed, and invested in the production of e-cigarettes. One of the companies to do so was Japan Tobacco International who bought a portion of Ploom, a start-up based in Silicon Valley, who produced a loose-leaf vaporizer.[1] E-cigarettes were also a gift to the emerging marijuana industry. Here was a device that could be used discreetly and without the offensive stench and exposure to marijuana smoke. These products were rapidly adopted by a segment of the public, prior to approval coming from the US FDA or Health Canada.

Rick Stevens, a former marketing executive, with 30 years in the tobacco industry, is the inventor and co-founder of JuJu Joints.[2] JuJu Joints, also referred to as e-joints, can contain 250 milligrams of cannabis oil.[2] They are also reported to contain propylene glycol, a chemical used to absorb water in foods and cosmetic products.[2] Suchitra Krishnan-Sarin, an associate professor of psychiatry at Yale University School of Medicine told *The New York Times* that it is not known what the effects of inhaling constant doses of this agent.[2]

Findings from *The National Youth Survey* show that the percentage of high school students, who reported "ever-using" an e-cigarette, rose from 4.7% in 2011 to 10% in 2012. In 2012 more than 1.78 million middle and high school students nationwide had tried e-cigarettes.[3]

"It's not surprising that more kids are using e-cigarettes and being poisoned by them as e-cigarettes are being marketed in ways that appeal to kids and sold in child-friendly flavors and colors. E-cigarettes have been marketed using the same tactics long used to market regular cigarettes to kids, including celebrity endorsements, slick TV and magazine ads, and sponsorships of race cars and concerns. Despite the fact that nicotine is toxic, nicotine liquids used in e-cigarettes are sold in a rainbow of colors and flavors including 'vivid vanilla', 'cherry crush', 'chocolate', 'Jolly Rancher', 'Gummy Bear' and 'Bubble Gum'."[4] —Matthew L. Myers, *Campaign for Tobacco-Free Kids*

"About 90 percent of all smokers begin smoking as teenagers," said Tim McAfee MD. M.P.H., director of the CDC Office on Smoking and Health.[6] "We must keep our youth from experimenting or using any tobacco product. These dramatic increases suggest that developing strategies to prevent marketing, sales, and use of e-cigarettes among youth is critical."[6] —McAfee

The California Department of Public Health found the use of e-cigarettes by adults in the state doubled from 2012 to 2013.[7]

The Centers for Disease Control and Prevention on April 16, 2015 released the *Morbidity and Mortality Weekly Report,* that showed e-cigarette use among middle and high school students had tripled from 2013 to 2014.[8] Findings from the 2014 the *NationalYouth Tobacco Survey*, showed that the e-cigarette use, defined as use on at least one day in the past 30 days among high school students, increased from 4.5 % in 2013 to 13.4 % in 2014. Among middle school students, e-cigarette use more than tripled from 1.1% in 2013 to 3.9% in 2014—with 120,000 to 450,000 students becoming customers. This was the first time since the survey started collecting data on e-cigarettes in 2011, that e-cigarette use had surpassed use of every other tobacco product overall.[9]

"We want parents to know that nicotine is dangerous to kids at any age, whether it's an e-cigarette, hookah, cigarette or cigar. Adolescence is a critical time for brain development. Nicotine exposure at a young age may cause lasting harm to brain development, promote addiction, and lead to sustained tobacco use," said the CDC Director.[6]

Data released in January 2015, from the American Association of Poison Control Centers, showed that poisoning incidents involving e-cigarettes and liquid nicotine jumped by 156% in one year, increasing more than 14 fold since 2011.[10] More than half the calls involved a child under the age of six, and one child died after ingesting liquid nicotine.[11],[12] Concern about the lack of scientific data on e-cigarettes and the growing popularity of these devices, caused a number of state and local governments to prohibit their use in public places. The Los Angeles City Council banned the use of electronic cigarettes in the workplace, in restaurants and in many public places, bringing their position on the public risk of e-cigarettes in line with the cities of New York along with Chicago.

E-cigarette Vapor can contain high concentrations of form-aldehyde.[13] "Vapor produced by e-cigarettes can contain form-aldehyde at levels five to 15 times higher than regular cigarettes, a new study finds. Formaldehyde is a known carcinogen."[14] —*Partnership News*. Another study, published by the *New England Journal of Medicine*, found that e-cigarette users who operate the devices at a high voltage are inhaling formaldehyde, and that the lifetime cancer risk of long-term "vaping" with the carcinogen inhaled, is five times as high as the risk associated with long-term smoking.[15]

Youth are using e-cigarettes to vaporize hash oil and wax infused with THC, or to vaporize dried cannabis leaves.

"We know that second-hand e-cigarette aerosol is not harmless, and it's critical to protect our nation's youth from this preventable health risk," said Brian King, deputy director for research translation in CDC's Office on Smoking and Health and a co-author of a study, published in *JAMA Pediatrics* in 2017.[16]

E-cigarette use among young people is a growing concern with an increase of 900 % from 2011 to 2015 and the use of flavors known to be especially attractive to young consumers. "One example is diacetyl, which is known to produce the buttery flavor in popcorn, and studies have linked inhalation of diacetyl to a severe respiratory illness," said King.[16]

CDC current data shows that 25% of middle school and high school students are exposed to vapors.[16]

THE MARIJUANA INDUSTRY AND VAPORIZING   Andrew Marantz writing for *The New Yorker Magazine* in 2014, reported on a conversation between Rohan Marley and Brendan

Kennedy.[17] "At the Henley Vaporium, in Nolita, Marley (Rohan) sat the "e-cig bar" and browsed a menus of favors— *Stop and Frisk, Cereal Killa*. Justin Haber, the "vapologist" on duty, took apart an e-cigarette to show how it worked."

"Can you smoke anything you want out of that?" Kennedy (Brendan) asked. Haber stiffened. "Hypothetically, if you had the proper—why are you asking?"—"Don't worry, brother, Marley said. 'We're starting a company, selling the herb above-board. Called *Marley Natural*. I'm one of Bob's boys, you understand?"[17]

When e-cigarette industry leader *NJOY* first attempted to import the devices from China in 2009, the U.S. Food and Drug Administration directed U.S. Customs to block the shipments. *NJOY* sued and successfully argued in court that e-cigarettes are a "tobacco product," and pleaded that the FDA didn't have the power to regulate these products. When the FDA did receive that authority and was a few weeks away from issuing federal rules asserting such authority to act, *NJOY* argued that its products were "smoking cessation devices" that did not contain tobacco and therefore should not be deemed a tobacco product under state or federal laws.[18] "And now that it's more convenient not to be, the same exact forces are out there making the opposite argument," said Stanton Glantz, Director of the Center for Tobacco Control Research and Education at the University of California, San Francisco.[18]

E-cigarettes have been promoted as a harm reduction strategy for smokers who are unable or unwilling to quit. A study by researchers at the University of California, San Francisco challenges the value and efficacy of e-cigarettes as a nicotine cessation device.[19]

VAPORIZING An increasingly popular way of using cannabis is with the use of vaporizers. Lower temperature vaporization of cannabis has been postulated as safer than smoking, but whether vaporizing cannabis is a safer alternative to smoking remains uncertain, as the reduction in toxic smoke components needs to be weighed against the hazards of acute intoxication and long-term consequences.

Philip Morris International reportedly spent $2 billion investing in new technology for their new *iQOS*, a device that is similar to an e-cigarette.[20] Developers claim the device delivers tobacco at one-third the temperature of regular burned cigarettes and therefore reduces the harm caused by the exposure to dangerous compounds.[20]

The holders of trademark licenses for brands, like *Girl Scout Cookies* and *Tootsie Rolls*, have formally objected to the brazen use of their iconic names for the promotion and branding of e-cigarettes.[21] In 2014 General Mills Inc., Girl Scouts of the USA and Tootsie Roll Industries issued cease-and-desist letters to makers of flavored nicotine liquids used in e-cigarettes.[22,23,24] "Using the *Thin Mint* name—which is synonymous with Girl Scouts and everything we do to enrich the lives of girls—to market e-cigarettes to youth is deceitful and shameless,[25]" Girl Scouts spokeswoman Kelly Parisi told *Associated Press*.

In January of 2017, *KTNV*, a news outlet in Nevada, reported on parents raising concerns over the use of the trademark name of *Girl Scout Cookies* to brand and market marijuana products.[26] The use of the name of *Girl Scout Cookies* has become an issue in other states. In California a dispensary was issued a cease and desist letter, to which they complied by removing the products bearing the name from their shelves.[27]

Canvasing a variety of online marijuana retailers, the Girl Scout name continues to be used in both Canada and the United States as of 2017.[28,29]

22. The Fight with Science

The medical evidence of the harm caused by tobacco products had been accumulating for approximately two centuries before it became widely acknowledged. The early science reported a caution for concern in relation to cancers of the lip and mouth, and then in relation to vascular disease and lung cancer.[1] Numerous case-control studies relating smoking, particularly of cigarettes, to the development of lung cancer were published in 1950, notable the work of Richard Doll in the United Kingdom and other studies in the United States.[2]

In 1950, the *Journal of the American Medical Association* published Ernest L.Wynder and Dr. (M.D.) Evarts A. Graham's *Tobacco Smoking as a Possible Etiologic Factor in Bronchiogenic Carcinoma: A Study of 684 Proven Cases.*[3] Wynder and Graham's retrospective study was not the first to link smoking and cancer, but its sophisticated design, impressive population size, and unambiguous findings established the need for further research. During the next decade, hundreds of reports were published linking cancer and smoking, including large prospective studies, pathologic, and animal investigations. The *Wynder/Graham Study* convinced many doctors that the health risks of smoking needed to be taken serious.

Many doctors would give up smoking, including Graham, who quit in 1952. Graham died in 1957 from lung cancer. He had been a heavy smoker.

The article *Cancer by the Carton,* originally written by Roy Norr for *The Christian Record,* was reprinted in a condensed format in the highly popular *Reader's Digest* edition of December of 1952. The size of the readership of *Reader's Digest* and the information provided by the article was taken as a serious threat by the tobacco industry. *The Frank Statement* advertisement was placed in 400 newspapers across America, and was the industry's response to their growing concern that their industry could be hurt by negative publicity.

The Frank Statement of 1954 was the tobacco industry's attempt to downplay the significance of the science that had emerged in the early 1950's. In their ad, they announced that the tobacco industry did not believe tobacco products to be injurious to human health.[4] The sponsors of the ad included, The American Tobacco Company, Benson and Hedges, Bright Belt Warehouse Association, Brown and Williamson Tobacco Corporation, Burley Auction Warehouse, Burley Tobacco Growers Cooperative Association, Larus and Brother Company Inc., P. Lorillard Company, Maryland Tobacco Growers Association, Philip Morris and Co. Ltd, RJ Reynolds Tobacco Company, Stephano Brothers Inc., Tobacco Associates, Inc. United States Tobacco Company. The list of sponsors also included the names of the CEO and principals for each entity.[4]

The 1954 industry ad was filed as a document in the Minnesota tobacco trials of 1994-1998. Judge Kenneth Fitzpatrick instructed members of the jury that they should assume in their deliberations a "special duty" by the industry, for allowing the publication of the *Frank* advert, and that it would be the juror's decision as to whether or not the sponsors of the ad fulfilled that duty. The jury found against the tobacco industry.[5] *The Frank Statement* is available online.[6]

In 1957, Surgeon General Leroy E. Burney declared it the official position of the US Public Health Service that the evidence pointed to a causal relationship between smoking and lung cancer.[7]

In June 1961, the American Cancer Society, the American Heart Association, the National Tuberculosis Association, and the American Public Health Association addressed a letter to President John F. Kennedy, in which they called for a national commission on smoking, dedicated to "seeking a solution to this health problem that would interfere least with the freedom of industry or the happiness of individuals".[8] The White House responded in 1962, after further evidence was provided by a highly publicized study on cigarette smoking released by the Royal College of Physicians, London, England.[9,10]

On June 7, 1962, Surgeon General Luther L. Terry announced that he would convene a committee of experts to conduct a comprehensive review of the scientific literature on the smoking and health question. Between November 1962 and January 1964, more than 7,000 scientific articles where scrutinized. By January 1964, Surgeon General Luther L. Terry, issued *Smoking and Health: Report of the Advisory Committee to the Surgeon General*, which held cigarette smoking responsible for a 70% increase in the mortality rate of (male) smokers over (male) non-smokers.[11] Women were not part of the study.

The commission's report released in January of 1964 made front page news and was a lead story on many radio and television station in the United States, and was broadcasted around the world. The public was in possession of the science and alerted to the serious links between smoking and lung cancer, coronary heart disease and other conditions.

Research on smoking tobacco products, conducted on data collected between 1997 and 2004 found that the disease risks from cigarette smoking increased over most of the twentieth century in the United States, as successive generations of first male and then female smokers began smoking at progressively earlier ages.[12]

In a 2013 editorial in *The New England Journal of Medicine*, Steven A. Schroeder, M.D. wrote that the hazard ratios for lung-cancer mortality were "staggering"; 17.8% for female smokers and 14.6% for male smokers. He also stated that the risk of death for women who smoke was 50% higher than the estimates reported in the 1980s.[13] Changes in how cigarettes had come to be manufactured, with perforated filters, more porous paper, that allowed for deeper inhalation of nicotine, along with other factors such as a change in tobacco blends may have made smoking more rather than less dangerous over time.

THE DEATH OF JOE CAMEL   Joe Camel was introduced in 1987, over twenty years after the Surgeon General had made his cautionary public statements. In five years, the annual sales of Camel cigarettes to teenagers rose from $6 million to $470 million.[14] In 1988, the *US Surgeon General's Report* concluded that nicotine was an addictive similar to heroin.[15] How Joe Camel ever came to the light of day let alone was front and centre in full neon in New York's Time Square in the 1980s is truly stupefying, given the warnings associated with the use of tobacco products that were widely publicized from the mid 1960's onward.

THE TOBACCO MASTER SETTLEMENT AGREEMENT (MSA)

In 1988, the first successful wrongful harm lawsuit of a smoker against a tobacco giant concluded. It would take another ten years before Joe Camel was forced off the shelf and dismantled from Times Square by the United States Government. The MSA was signed in 1998, by the four largest American tobacco companies and the attorney generals of 46 states. The tobacco industry was forced to compensate the American nation for a portion of the health care costs associated with caring for people with smoking-related diseases. The amount was to be paid over a 25-year period and amounted to more than $240 billion.[16]

The MSA said that a sizeable portion of the settlement funds were to be used by state government agencies to run the public health prevention programs. Financial reports from 2012, show individual states had cut their funding for tobacco prevention and cessation programs to levels not seen since the first settlement funds were paid out.[17] The states in fiscal year 2012 collected $25.6 billion in revenue from the tobacco settlement and tobacco taxes, but spent only 1.8% of it—$456.7 million—on programs to prevent kids from smoking and helping smokers quit.[17] The states spent less than two cents of every dollar in tobacco revenue to fight tobacco use.[17]

Under the MSA, the tobacco industry was also forced to stop certain tobacco marketing practices, including the use of cartoon characters in the promotion of their products. It was established not only that young children were attracted to the images of Joe Camel, but that this exposure primed children for tobacco use in their youth.[18]

An ongoing international campaign seeks to restrict the depiction of smoking in films viewed by the young. The World Health Organization first spotlighted the issue in 2003 on *World No-Tobacco Day*.

Jonathan Samet, writing for *Tobacco Control* concluded: "The evidence continues to support the case that exposure to smoking in movies is one specifically remediable determinant of initiation, and a determinant with global reach."[19]

RETALIATION In 1999, the year following the *MSA* placing restrictions on certain forms of advertising, the major cigarette companies spent a record $8.4 billion on marketing.[20]

According to research produced in 2007 through Harvard School of Public Health, the amount of nicotine that smokers consumed per cigarette, regardless of brand or manufacturer, increased an average of 1.6% per year from 1998 to 2004.[21] The Harvard study claims, that cigarette manufacturers had intentionally increased their products' nicotine levels to produce a more addictive product. The research found that nicotine levels in cigarettes from all major manufacturers increased by 11% from 1997 and 2005. The tobacco industry dismissed these findings outright.[21]

Following the *MSA*, the four principal tobacco companies raised their prices more than 45 cents per pack.[22] The costs of the *MSA*, as predicted by critics of the settlement, were passed on to the consumer.

In 2012, the Australian government implemented a public policy for all tobacco products to be sold in olive-coloured, plain packaging with graphic health warnings. Uruguay and Australia have been engaged in legal battles with tobacco companies, over laws requiring graphic health warning labels or standard packaging for cigarettes without logos. The tobacco companies have countered the claim and are hold the position that tobacco-control policies violate international trade agreements and World Trade Organization rules.[23]

In 2013, Imperial Tobacco introduced a new line of cigarettes.[24] The company hired prominent artists from around the world to make every detail an inspiring piece of art and turn a habitual cigarette package into a unique masterpiece of contemporary art.

Former New York Mayor Michael Bloomberg and Microsoft Corp. co-founder Bill Gates launched a fund to help low and middle-income countries fight often tedious and expensive legal battles with the tobacco industry. *The Anti-Tobacco Trade Litigation Fund*, backed by $4 million from Bloomberg Philanthropies and the Bill & Melinda Gates Foundation, was announced at the 16th World Conference on Tobacco or Health in Abu Dhabi, United Arab Emirates in 2015.[25]

The Trans-Pacific Partnership Agreement (TPP) concluded with built-in protections to prevent private corporations from suing governments over anti-tobacco regulations. "The victory comes after years of pressure from a vast coalition of health groups and pro-health legislators, including Action on Smoking and Health (ASH), to protect the right of governments to regulate tobacco without fear of expensive lawsuits....A small number of pro-tobacco legislators vowed to try to kill the Agreement over the tobacco carve-out."[26]
—*Tobacco Carve-Out in TPP,* (2015)

The tobacco industry has a long history of using costly litigation to scaring off opponents, who wish to limit their corporate behavior. The TPP was the first major trade agreement to carve-out protections for tobacco measures. In January 2017 the USA government announced it would withdraw from supporting the TPP Agreement.

Decades after the settlement of the American government with the tobacco industry, Canada has not resolved the issue of damage. The pursuit is ongoing, with the potential claim being in excess of $110 billion.[27]

In the United States, the warnings on the lateral side of cigarette packages have not been changed since 1985.[28] On October 7, 2016, public health and medical groups and several individual pediatricians filed a suit, in federal court in Boston, to force the U.S. Food and Drug Administration (FDA) to issue a final rule requiring graphic health warnings on cigarette packs and advertising, as mandated by a 2009 federal law.

The 2009 *Family Smoking Prevention and Tobacco Control Act* required graphic warnings covering the top half of the front and back of cigarette packs and 20 percent of cigarette advertising. The FDA had until June 22, 2011, to issue a final rule requiring such warnings. The graphic warnings required by the FDA were struck down in August 2012 by a three-judge panel of the U.S. Court of Appeals for the D.C. Circuit, which ruled 2-1 that the proposed warnings violated the *First Amendment*.[28] Ruling in March of 2012, the U.S. Court of Appeals for the Sixth Circuit upheld the law's requirement for graphic warnings, finding that this provision did not violate the *First Amendment*.[28] The court found the warnings "are reasonably related to the government's interest

in preventing consumer deception and are therefore constitutional."[29] The U.S. Supreme Court declined to hear a tobacco
industry appeal of the ruling. The lawsuit filed in October
of 2016, alleged that the FDA's failure to issue a new rule
requiring graphic warnings is "agency action unlawfully withheld" and seeks a court order requiring the FDA to proceed
with a new set of graphic warnings. The lawsuit was filed in
the U.S. District Court for the District of Massachusetts. The
graphic warnings had been mandated by a large, bipartisan
majority of Congress, who were convinced of the need for the
warnings. A study published in 2013, found that after Canada
mandated graphic warnings, smoking rates declined 3 to 5
percentage points. The study estimated that if the United
States had adopted the warnings in 2012, within a year 5.3
million to 8.6 million fewer people would be smoking.[29]

The final report of the Canadian Task Force on cannabis
legalization and regulation of November 30, 2016 concluded:
"In designing a system for the regulation of cannabis, we are
creating a new industry. As with other industries, this new cannabis industry will seek to increase its profits and expand its
market, including through the use of advertising and promotion. Because of the risks discussed earlier in this chapter, regulation aims to discourage use among youth and ensure that
only evidence-informed information is provided to adults.
Restrictions on advertising, promotion and related activities
are therefore necessary."[30]

The report recommended that the federal government:
"Apply comprehensive restrictions to the advertising and
promotion of cannabis and related merchandise by any
means, including sponsorship, endorsements and branding,

similar to the restrictions on promotion of tobacco product. Allow limited promotion in areas accessible by adults, similar to those restrictions under the *Tobacco Act*. Require plain packaging for cannabis products that allows the following information on packages: company name, strain name, price, amounts of THC and CBD and warnings and other labelling requirements. Impose strict sanctions on false or misleading promotion as well as promotion that encourages excessive consumption, where it is allowed. Require that any therapeutic claims made in advertising conform to applicable legislation. Resource and enable the detection and enforcement of advertising and marketing violations, including via traditional and social media."[30]

"In designing a system for the regulation of cannabis, we are creating a new industry."[30] —Canadian Task Force.

For years, illegal marijuana stores have been open for business across Canada, supported by web-based sales, billboards, and with store-front neon advertising and brick and mortar main-street operations. Advertising narcotics is violation of the *Criminal Code* of Canada. The fines are heavy, ranging from prison time to multi-million dollar fines.

Controlling the advertising, promotion and influence of the tobacco industry as well as the rapidly expanding marijuana industry in the age of social media and internet sales and marketing could very well be unattainable.

One of the world's largest tobacco producers elected to remove the word "tobacco" from their name in 2016.[31] The monolithic entity is now to be known as Imperial Brands. In June of 2017 Imperial Brands hired Simon Langelier to join the board as a non-executive director.[32] Mr. Langelier spent 30 years working at tobacco rival Philip Morris and he is chairman of PharmaCielo, a Canadian company that supplies cannabis oil for medical purposes.[32]

23. The Truth

THE TOBACCO TRUTH CAMPAIGN   Successful marketing slogans have three components; they consist of four words or less, are memorable and they are believable. The most successful counter-tobacco campaign, ever to have run in America, brought the conversation to one word—the word truth.

The Florida Tobacco Pilot Program, ran from 1998 to 1999, under the leadership of the Governor of Florida, Lawton Chiles, with Chuck Wolfe as the architect of the initiative.[1] The campaign sought to engage the youth sector with the slogan; *truth, a generation united against tobacco.*[1] They launched a $25 million advertising campaign, with television commercials, billboards, print ads and posters. The ads re-framed the tobacco-conversation, and struck out against corporate greed, manipulation and deceit.

Turning negative into positive: public health mass media campaigns and negative advertising, written by D.E. Apollonio, R.E. Malone, in November 2008, (*Oxford Press*) argues: "When corporate disease vectors such as the tobacco industry control interpretive voice through advertising and promotion, public health-oriented negative advertising can promote alternative interpretations that disrupt corporate messages. This reframing may be the most effective long-term strategy in controlling complex public health problems that have multiple causes."[2]

Truth (stylized as truth), is an ongoing national campaign in America. In August 2014, *truth* launched *Finish It,* a redesigned campaign encouraging youth to be the generation that ends smoking.[3]

Tobacco industry denormalization (TID) is a tobacco control strategy that illustrates how the tobacco industry operates outside the norms of legitimate corporate behaviour.

"Tobacco industry de-normalization is a public health strategy the places the responsibility for the tobacco epidemic where it belongs, on corporate misbehavior rather than on individual misjudgement. TID puts a spotlight on corporate fraud, negligence and failure to warn rather than on teenage miscalculation of the risks of addiction or on the failure of youth to recognize that they are the targets of predatory marketing by adults. The TID strategy shows the public that the industry and its products are not legitimate, or normal, and they warrant marginalization."[4] —Garfield Mahood, the founder of the Non-smoker's Rights Association of Canada

THE TOBACCO INDUSTRY'S RESPONSE TO TID "Industry members enjoy a constitutional right not to be subjected to denormalization policies or tactics."[5] —Rothmans Inc. "Such denormalization is the antithesis of the freedom embodied in the *Charter (Canadian Charter of Rights and Freedoms)* and is entirely incompatible with individual liberties."[6] —Imperial Tobacco

A Health Canada statement on TID reads: "Traditionally, anti-smoking social marketing efforts have been directed at making smoking a less socially acceptable behaviour without blaming the victim. Denormalization, in the context of social behaviour, aims to change attitudes toward what is generally regarded as normal or acceptable behaviour, including through social marketing. When attitudes change, behaviour will also change because humans generally want to act in ways that are acceptable to others. There is clearly scope to consider further behavioural denormalization, particularly where it focuses on the consequences for others, rather than just the person smoking: Working to discourage smoking in enclosed public or private spaces where others could be affected by second-hand smoke, including children in the home; Working to discourage smoking by and around pregnant women.

However, consideration can be given to approaches to denormalization that go beyond the individual. Another possibility is promoting greater awareness of the effects of second-hand smoke on non-smokers' health, and to provide appropriate support for increased smoke-free areas. Additional possibilities lie in creating greater awareness of the extent of criminal sales to children (50 million criminal sales per year), and the role the retail sector plays in displaying, promoting and selling cigarettes to children.

Rather than 'smoking', increased focus can be placed on use of 'tobacco products' and their effects. Denormalization activity can be employed to expose the way the tobacco industry operates and shifting the focus to tobacco products versus "smoking". Denormalization could help build public support for tobacco control measures and public concern about the tobacco industry.

This type of denormalization activity can include: Deglamorizing the use of tobacco products; Combatting myths about tobacco products (for example, that light and mild products are safer or can help you quit); Drawing attention to the size and impact of tobacco industry advertising budgets, and the nature of their promotional activities; Drawing attention to the role of other industries and organizations in supporting the promotion and sale of tobacco.

Denormalization activities are important because they may help develop a set of values and behaviours that bring the whole community together to reinforce desirable behaviour and attitudes. It can help make tobacco use an issue of community concern, rather than just an issue for those using the products. Secondly, it can help ensure that people behave in appropriate ways--including making efforts to quit--without the need for a lot of policing or enforcement. Thirdly, it can help generate support for Government and broader defence of public health policy in the face of industry challenges.

Examples of possible benefits of denormalization in the context of tobacco, could include: Any attempt to sell cigarettes to minors would be discouraged by attention from other shoppers; People using tobacco products in places where others were affected by smoke would attract adverse attention; Canadians would accept health advice relating to tobacco use and cessation from credible sources only; and Canadians would be sensitized to promotional techniques, particularly where they influence children.

Corporations currently engaged in partnerships with tobacco companies (i.e., Banks, newspapers, advertisers, governments and other co-sponsors) would disengage from supporting tobacco promotion and sales. Governments would gradually cease their promotion and support of tobacco-promoting events (i.e., Co-sponsored festivals) and the promotion of tobacco production and sale (i.e., Trade missions which encourage tobacco exports)."[7]

The United Nations Human Rights Council endorses the *UN Guiding Principles on Business and Human Rights* (*UNGP*) that apply to all companies. According to the UNGPs all companies must avoid causing or contributing to adverse impacts on human rights.[8] The production of tobacco is irreconcilable with the human right to health. The UNGPs has called for and requires the cessation of the production and marketing of tobacco products.[9] The UNGP is the authoritative global standard for addressing human right abuses by companies. These are global human rights standards which apply equally to all countries, the U.S. and Canada included.

In May of 2017, Philip Morris International launched a manifesto on their website. The front page banner reads: *Designing a Smoke-Free Future. How long will the world's leading cigarette company be in the cigarette business?*[10] It is a question that requires an answer, from a co-ordinated international voice.

PIRATE CAPITALISM In 1992, 7% of Russian women smoked cigarettes and the percentage would more than double over the subsequent decade.[11] Over the same time period, the number of Russian men who smoked rose only 5%, from 57% to 63%.[11] The 2009, *Global Adult Tobacco Survey*, shows the smoking rate for Russian women (ages 19-24), had risen to an estimated 37.9%.[12]

A study published in *Tobacco Control* credits the rise in consumption by Russian women on the privatization of the previously state owned tobacco industry, and the arrival of the international tobacco companies.[13] Russia saw an influx of approximately $1.7 US billion between 1992 and 2000, to gain a 60% portion of the privatized tobacco market in Russia.[13]

"There can be no doubt that the marketing tactics of Philip Morris, British American Tobacco and the like directly underpin this massive increase in smoking that spells disaster for health in Russia," said Dr. Anna Gilmore from the School for Health at the University of Bath.[14]

"Under pressure at home for marketing an addictive and deadly product, domestic sales were shrinking. It was a dilemma Bain and Romney knew well, having worked extensively on behalf of Philip Morris in the U.S. beginning in 1990. In 1992, Bain approached British American Tobacco (the international conglomerate behind Kool, Lucky Strike, Pall Mall and Benson & Hedges) offering a lucrative partnership in Russia. It worked."[15] —*The Huffington Post* (USA)

"Between 1975 and 1994, overall cigarette sales in the United States declined by more than 20 percent (from 607.2 to 485 billion cigarettes). During the same period, production of American cigarettes rose by 11 percent."[16] —*The Cigarette Century.*

FOLLOWING BIG TOBACCO A rising concern, now coming from the international drug prevention community, is whether or not "Big Marijuana", under the provisions of free trade agreements, will be able to advance marijuana products to the world population. Selling marijuana products, known to be hallucinogens, addictive and harmful to the mind and body, into regions that do not have restrictions in place on promotion, nor adequate public health campaigns, is viewed as a significant threat to world health. That marijuana products could be pushed on young populations, wholly ill-equipped to fight off the industry's advances, demands serious consideration.

In a letter, addressed to the Canadian Prime Minister, Justin Trudeau on August 26, 2016, Eze Eluchie, LL.B., LL.M, BL., Executive Director of the PADDI Foundation (People against Drug Dependence and Ignorance) and board member of the World Federation against Drugs (WFAD) wrote: "With benefit of hindsight from the continuing dire consequences to the Africa region resulting from the activities of Multinational Tobacco Conglomerates (the tobacco industry), we are particularly concerned that with the combination of the current efforts of the Government of Canada to internationalize the legalization and commercialization of marijuana and the protections accorded "legal and "commercial" products under the World Trade Organizations statuses and protocols, the African region stands the risk of being overwhelmed and serving as the ultimate dumping ground for the 'legalized and commercialized marijuana products.' When this scenario is added to the African regions already worrisome public health and social security environment, our worries will be better appreciated."[17]

A letter was dispatched on August 30, 2016 to the Prime Minister of Canada from the International President of the World Federation against Drugs, Sven-Olov Carlsson. Mr. Carlsson wrote: "WFAD is a global organization, but the majority of our member organizations are based in the global south, and their testimonies and experience is clear. The legalization of drugs in the west is influencing also the youth in, for example, the slums of Nairobi but also the attitudes towards legalization in the general population.

Rich countries are failing to find the resources to address their drug problems and care for their children and their poor, how can we expect that less developed countries will find the resources. The world's poorest communities are the most vulnerable to the harms of drug use and trade. They will not be able to regulate the marketing or collect taxes from drug sales, simply because there are not taxes to collect."[18]

"I'm not sure I could work in the tobacco industry. I'm not sure I could work in the alcohol industry. But we eventually got comfortable with that moral question and in fact, you know today, having talked to so many patients and physicians and talked to so many activists who are interested in individual civil liberties or patient rights, you know we feel this moral imperative to succeed."[19] —Brendan Kennedy, Privateer Holdings.

In May of 2016, Tilray announced they were launching a cross country motor tour to match prospect marijuana customers with doctors.[20] A company media release said doctors would be able to sign people up and "prescribe on the spot".[20] Philippe Lucas, VP of patient research and advocacy for Tilray, told the Canadian media that the company was responding to patients who were having trouble finding a supportive physician to access marijuana.[20] The photo that accompanied the article showed an airstream trailer decked out with large lettering that read: "Mobile Cannabis Clinic, sponsored by Tilray."

In June of 2016, the Canadian media reported that Health Canada had granted an export license to Tilray, for the exportation of marijuana products for medical purposes to Croatia. Tilray President, Brendan Kennedy told the Canadian media that the company was the first of the Canadian licensed and legal producers to ship marijuana products for medical purposes outside of Canada.[21] More companies would follow, with a total of four holding export licenses by mid-2017. Kennedy also spoke of their interest in global expansion.[21] Tilray received the approval to export and distribute medi-pot into Chile in 2017.[22] With this development the company announced that it now had a presence on four continents.[23]

In July of 2016, a *Globe and Mail* headline read: "Canada's medical pot companies aim to grow export business".[24] Canopy Growth Corp, another Canadian licensed and legal producer, had announced that it would soon begin to sell dried canna-bis in pharmacies across Germany.[24] They had been granted an export license from Health Canada. The company plan was to open a factory in Germany, as it was expected Germany would move to legalize marijuana for medical purposes in the coming year. Germany legalized marijuana for medical purposes in the spring of 2017.

In March of 2017, the Ministry of Health of the Government of Canada released a document: *Seizing the opportunity: the future of tobacco control in Canada*. The document suggested, that in partnership with all Canadians, the Government was willing to take action to drive down tobacco product use in Canada to less than 5% by 2035.[25] The Canadian government was pre-paring to introduce new legislation in the Canadian House of Commons in the next month that would make smoked mari-juana products legal, albeit with restrictions.

Studies released from The National Institute of Drug Abuse (NIDA) found that using marijuana can lead to a higher likelihood of nicotine addiction due to changes in the brain.[26] "While tobacco use does commonly precede marijuana use, we propose that marijuana may be a "gateway drug" to tobacco

smoking. Our research with university students is suggesting that cigarette-smoking initiation often follows or coincides with marijuana. Pre-venting the process of learning how to smoke should be a primary goal of future prevention efforts, which aim to decrease ALL smoking behaviors, especially in youth."[27]
—*Marijuana and Tobacco: A Major Connection? Journal of Addiction Diseases,* (2003)

24. The Piper's Tune

COLD TURKEY Nicotine replacement therapy products (NRT) were introduced to the American market through the use of the promotional slogan, "Don't Go Cold Turkey", which was attached to a national campaign organized by Glaxton Smith Pharmaceuticals.[1] The campaign aimed to convince people who smoked, to not attempt spontaneous abstinence. The effect of this carefully crafted messaging was that it reinforced the belief that quitting smoking was hard to do.

The following excerpts from Chapman S, MacKenzie R (2010), *The Global Research Neglect of Unassisted Smoking Cessation: Causes and Consequences*, outline the incredible story behind smoking cessation and NRT: "Today, unassisted cessation continues to lead the next most successful method NRT by a wide margin. Yet, paradoxically, the tobacco control community treats this information as if it was somehow irresponsible or subversive and ignores the potential policy implications of studying self-quitters. Unassisted cessation is seldom emphasised in advice to smokers.... Because of these prevalent attitudes, smoking cessation is becoming increasingly pathologised, a development that risks distortion of public awareness of how most smokers quit to the obvious benefit of pharmaceutical companies. Furthermore, the cessation research literature is preoccupied with the difficulty of stopping. Notably, however, in the rare literature that has bothered to ask, many ex-smokers recall stopping as less traumatic than anticipated. For example, in a large British study of ex-smokers in the 1980s, before the advent of pharmacotherapy, 53% of the ex-smokers said that it was 'not at all difficult' to stop, 27% said it was 'fairly difficult', and the remainder found it 'very difficult'.

The availability of pharmaceutical industry research funding—often provided without the lengthy processes of open tender or independent peer review—can be highly attractive to researchers. Furthermore, it is often observed that 'research follows the money,' with scientists being drawn to well-funded research areas....This greater availability of funding for certain sorts of research produces a distorted research emphasis on pharmacotherapy that, when combined with the industry's formidable public relations abilities and direct-to-consumer advertising, concentrates both scientific and public discourse on cessation around assisted pharmacotherapy.... Meanwhile, the massive decline in smoking that occurred before the advent of cessation treatment is often forgotten....Other than the first small pack warnings that appeared from 1966 in the USA, this effect occurred without any elements of today's comprehensive approaches to tobacco control.

The public is often advised that assistance at least doubles cessation rates. But while the clinical trial literature consistently shows higher quit rates from assisted than unassisted cessation, population studies show the opposite."[1]

Multiple attempts at "cold turkey, not a single attempt, is how the majority of people quit smoking. In 1986, the American

Cancer Society reported: "Over 90% of the estimated 37 million people who have stopped smoking in this country since the Surgeon General's first report linking smoking to cancer have done so unaided."[2]

The manufacturers of NRT products do not make claims about long-term abstinence—they state that the products are designed to assist with withdrawal symptoms.[3] In 2011, the Harvard School of Public Health released the following information: "Nicotine replacement therapy (NRT) designed to help people stop smoking, specifically nicotine patches and nicotine gum, do not appear to be effective in helping smokers quit long-term, even when combined with smoking cessation counseling, according to a new study by researchers at Harvard School of Public Health and the University of Massachusetts Boston.[4] The researchers found no difference in relapse rates among those who used NRT for more than six weeks, with or without professional counseling. No difference in quitting success with use of NRT was found for either heavy or light smokers. The study demonstrates that using NRT is no more effective in helping people stop smoking cigarettes in the long-term than quitting unaided."[4]

The Public Health Service, a division of the USA Department of Health and Human Services in 2000, released a set of guidelines calling for smokers to use nicotine patches, gums and other pharmaceutical aids to quit, with a few exceptions such as pregnant women.[5] The government of British Columbia, Canada is but one entity that continues to contribute tens of millions of dollars annually, to provide free nicotine replacement therapy to people who are desirous of butting out and are considered "hardened" past the hope of abstinence.[6,7]

SOLD INTO ADDICTION   Individuals who smoke cigarettes commonly come to believe that the use of tobacco/nicotine products offers genuine relaxation. A psychological and or physical sense of calm is easily confused with the relief from the cycle of drug use and the agitation experienced in a state of withdrawal. Understanding that nicotine is a physical stimulant and not a relaxant, and what the user is experiencing is drug addiction and not physical relaxation, is helpful in assisting individuals to get off tobacco. Challenging perceived benefits has proven to be transformational.[8]

Marketing, advertising, and peddling marijuana for medical purposes under the premise that these products can produce a beneficial emotional state is selling the psychological belief component of addiction.

The Oregonian editorial staff requested Leafly to review the search terms used by Oregon marijuana consumers for their pot preferences.[9] The top strains by consumer preference were listed as: *Blue Dream, Blackberry Kush, Jack Herer, Cinex, Blue Magoo, Sour Diesel, Girl Scout Cookies, Bubba Kush, OG Kush,* and *Trainwreck.*[9] *Blue Dream* was the most popular marijuana strain in Portland, *Trainwreck* in Eugene. *Blue Dream, Blackberry, KushBlue, Magoo Jack, Herer, Cinex, Obama, Kush, Scout Cookies* in Seattle.[9] Creativity was the most sought-after effect from marijuana use, followed by the other popular effects; happiness, euphoria, energy and relaxation.[9] The top conditions listed for why consumers in Oregon wanted marijuana included anxiety, attention deficit disorder, bipolar disorder, migraines and post-traumatic stress disorder.[9] The article did make note that none of the named effects were considered qualifying conditions for medical marijuana access.

ONWARD On July 13, 2017 *Reuters* reported that it had been discovered that Philip Morris International has been running a secretive campaign to block or weaken treaty provisions that aim to save millions of lives by curbing tobacco use.

Confidential corporate documents and interviews with current and former Philip Morris employees revealed an offensive campaign by the industry leaders covering the Americas to Africa to Asia. This is considered one of the largest tobacco industry leaks ever. *Reuters* announced they would be publishing some of the papers online and they provided the address; *The Philip Morris Files.*[10]

In the closing days of July 2017 the United States Government announced an intention to pursue limiting the level of nicotine potency in cigarettes. It was suggested that such a move could work to curb addiction to tobacco products. It is a step, however small in the right direction.

On October 4, 2017 The (UK) Daily Mail ran the following story: Smoking-cannabis-DOES-make-people-violent.[11] The research under discussion was Persistency of cannabis Use Predicts Violence following acute Psychiatric Discharge, conducted by scientists at the Centre de recherche de l'Institut Universitaire en Santé Mentale de Montréal, Montréal, QC, Canada, A Google search did not show any Canadian media covering the study.[12]

25. Twas4Kids

THE TWAS4KIDS PROJECT In 2012, I was afforded a voice in the tobacco prevention network when I edited and published a "smoke-free" edition of what is arguably the most famous poem in the English language. With a simple edit of a few words, and with a change in the illustrations, Santa, who had been a depicted as a smoker for close to 200 years, smoked no more. Gone were the twenty one words: "The stump of a pipe he held tight in his teeth, and the smoke it encircled this head like a wreath."

The 2012 edited version of Clement C. Moore's 1822 poem, *Twas the Night Before Christmas*, created a media stir upon its release, with a controversy playing out in the international media over whether the "smoking" edit was justified or constituted an act of censorship.

"Santa doesn't go around killing kids. He doesn't leave them bombs. I just think starting to rewrite and revise all of our history leads to something even more meaningless than even Disney," scoffed Alvin Schrader, a professor emeritus at the University of Alberta and convenor of the Canadian Library Association's Intellectual Freedom Advisory Committee.[1] "Although it's now in the public domain, there's something disturbing about modifying a classic," said educator Ms. de Vos. "What about those children who never get to hear the real thing? What if they become an adult and find out Santa used to be a smoker?"[1] "I think it is dreadful." said Professor Ann Curry, who along with Ms. De Vos teaches at the University of Alberta.[1] These comments appeared on the cover, and on page two of the *National Post* on September 19, 2012.

The American Library Association weighed in on the topic choosing to view the edit as censorship.[2] They expressed their strong objection on both *National Public Radio* (NPR) out of Los Angeles and on the national aired *CBC* radio show, *The Current Review*.[2, 3] The Deputy Director of the American Library Association told *CBC* reporter Laura Lynch in the broadcast: "It's still kind of an act of literary, uh.., uh...vandalism."[3]

The Cincinnati, Ohio legal firm of Wood Herron and Evans (LLP) was retained, to seek a retraction of and remediation for certain statements made by Deborah Caldwell-Smith, in her capacity as Deputy Director of the Office for Intellectual Freedom of the American Library Association. In a letter dated May 13, 2013, Stephen E. Gillen concludes: "The GSP (Grafton and Scratch Publishers) edition does not constitute an act of literary vandalism and, quite the contrary, represents an entirely legitimate approach to furthering a critical public health interest."[4]

The smoking-edit captured commentary on the *Colbert Report*, hosted by Stephen Colbert, was covered by *The Associated Press*, *The New York Post*, and hundreds of international media outlets.[5, 6, 7, 8] The media attention provided an opportunity to advocate for greater protective measures designed to guard young children from imagery and influences in popular culture that have been shown to normalize tobacco products. Did the project stop children from smoking down the line? That is impossible to answer. Readers were offered a smoke-free option, the project stimulated engagement, and shook up a measure of complacency on the public health issue of youth initiation to smoked products.

A SMOKE-FREE GENERATION   One thousand children in the UK, between the ages of 7 and 13, were polled on their attitudes toward parental smoking of tobacco by the British Department of Health in 2009.[9] Over half of the children said that their one wish for Christmas was for their parent(s) to quit smoking. Close to three quarters of children with a smoking parent, told the researchers they worried of their parent dying. Almost a third of children surveyed admitted to hiding their parent's cigarettes in an attempt to help them quit.[9]

The smoke-free edition of *Twas the Night Before Christmas* is for all children who worry about their loved ones who continue to smoke. *The Pied Pipers of Pot* aims to stimulate discussion over the very serious problem of children exposed to the use of marijuana products, including exposure in their homes to second hand and third hand smoke.

The material that forms this book was taken from my notes as a child-rights activists. Having lived through the pot era of the 1970s and 1980s, as first a high-school student and later at university, I was able to bring my direct personal experience to the present marijuana discussions. Many of my generation participated as marijuana consumers in their youth. I chose not to purchase illicit drugs. I did not want to give money to black market operators. The decision was that simple.

All of us live with a shared social contract which provides for help if need be. The caveat to the arrangement is clear; "wear the seatbelt"—"reject the use of narcotics"—"do not support illegal operations". Roughly 10% of the population in North American has been willing to break the law, and purchase drugs from illicit sources. Turning illicit dealers into legitimate members of the merchant class does not adequately address the issue. However, deciding to put down the drugs would go a long way.

Offer children the science on marijuana products and they are best equipped to protect themselves from the solicitations made by the peddlers of addictive products. Not all of life's lessons must be learned by direct personal experimentation, or through observing damage experienced by others. Prevention does work when implemented. The goal of prohibition is achievable and it starts with reducing demand by one, and sharing that success with others.

To prepare for the impending legalization of marijuana researchers from Montreal's Concordia University, reviewed three national surveys from Canada and the US as well as the scientific literature.[10] The researchers found that nearly all marijuana use in Canada begins in adolescence, with people who do not use marijuana before age 21 almost never going on to use it.[10]

Like most other researchers who have examined the health impacts of marijuana, they found the drug has harmful effects on both physical and mental health that persist even after use stops. They further stated that Canadian teenagers who start using before age 15; "will suffer for the rest of their lives even if they never use marijuana after the age of 21."[10] They reported that only five percent of Canadian teenagers perceive regular marijuana use to be a health hazard.[10]

A CROP poll conducted on behalf of *CBC*'s French-language network Radio-Canada, released in May of 2017, showed 40% of Quebecers were strongly or somewhat in favour of legalization when asked: "Are you in favour or against legalization of cannabis?"[11] The majority expressed their rejection of legalization and their lack of confidence in the promised benefits of legalization being put forth by the federal government.[11] Quebecers were much more pessimistic over the impending legalization of marijuana than Canadians in other regions of the country. The pollster offered several possible explanations for the divide in opinion including the aging of the Quebec population, but also the influence of the U.S. English speaking media that have exposed English Canadians to "much talk" of marijuana legalization. [11]

A driver was killed, along with two other passengers, ages 15 and 20, on a highway outside Lander, Wyoming.[12] The driver's cannabis by-product levels was 10 times higher than levels that mark impaired driving by the National Traffic Highway Safety Administration and Wyoming law. A fourth person who was involved in the accident was seriously injured.[12] The Coroner's office on writing a report on the case said it hopes awareness of the circumstances in the case will spur friends, families, and the public as a whole to take steps to safeguard against any person driving while impaired, whether by alcohol or any other substance.[12]

The madness has to end.

Index

You may also enjoy reading:

On Marijuana: A Powerful Examination of What Marijuana Means to Our Children, Our Communities and Our Future. Compiled by Pamela McColl, forward by Kevin Sabet Ph.D., and David Frum.

Baby and Me Tobacco Free—quitting smoking before a child comes into your life. Written by Laurie Adams and Pamela McColl. The book outlines the smoking cessation program created to reduce the burden of tobacco use for parents who are looking forward to starting a family and want to do so smoke-free.

Twas The Night Before Christmas edited by Santa Claus For The Benefit of Children of the 21st Century, Clement C. Moore. What *Kirkus Review* calls a legitimate editing of the reference to the pipe and wreath of smoke. Published in English, Spanish and French.

The Pied Piper of Hamelin is a Germany legend that portrays a piper, dressed in multicolored ("pied") clothing, who was a rat-catcher hired by the town to lure rats away with his magic pipe. When he was not paid for his work he retaliates by using his instrument's magical power on townspeople's children, leading them away as he had the rats.

Notes

Introduction

1. http://www.huffingtonpost.co.uk/paul-hayes/drug-policy-uk-untold-success-story_b_6098594. html

2. http://www.cnbc.com/2014/01/16/companies-woo-the-weed-crowd-with-artful-edgy-ads.html

3. http://www.abc.net.au/foreign/content/2014/s4027079.htm Cannabis Inc. Permission Granted Producer Suzanne Smith, Foreign Correspondent.

4. Johnston, L. D., O'Malley, P. M., Miech, R. A., Bachman, J. G., & Schulenberg, J. E. (2017). Monitoring the Future national survey results on drug use, 1975-2016: Overview, key findings on adolescent drug use. Ann Arbor: Institute for Social Research, The University of Michigan. Public domain.

5. Porath-Waller, A.J., Brown, J.E., Frigon, A.P., & Clark, H. (2013). What Canadian youth think about Cannabis. Ottawa, Ontario: Canadian Centre on Substance Abuse. 2013

6. http://www.ccsa.ca/Resource%20Library/CCSA-Canadian-Youth-Perceptions-on-Cannabis-Report-2017-en.pdf. 2016

7. http://www.unicef.ca/sites/default/files/imce_uploads/DISCOVER/OUR%20WORK/ADVOCACY/DOMESTIC/POLICY%20ADVOCACY/DOCS/unicef_rc_11_canadian_companion.pdf. Unicef 2013/IRC11 Stuck In The Middle

8. http://smartcolorado.org/permission Harrison Chamberlain

9. https://psychcentral.com/news/2013/05/27/parents-do-influence-teen-use-of-illicit-substances/55307.html

10. http://www.huffingtonpost.ca/entry/just-say-now-left-right-c_n_669043

   a) http://www.cbc.ca/news/canada/british-columbia/illegal-marijuana-dispensaries-not-a-priority-for-vancouver-police-chief-adam-palmer-1.3131817

   b) http://fortune.com/2014/08/02/leafly-new-york-times-full-page-advertisement/

11. http://www.seattletimes.com/nwshowcase/careers/the-case-for-eating-weed-at-work/

12. https://medicalxpress.com/news/2017-05-marijuana-tied-poorer-school.html

13. http://www.independent.co.uk/news/education/education-news/weed-marijuana-cannabis-use-linked-poor-school-performance-teenagers-study-exams-university-waterloo-a7730126. html a) PNAS Plus - Social Sciences - Psychological and Cognitive Sciences: Madeline H.

Meier, Avshalom Caspi, Antony Ambler, HonaLee Harrington, Renate Houts, Richard S. E. Keefe, Kay McDonald, Aimee Ward, Richie Poulton, and Terrie E. Moffitt. Persistent cannabis users show neuropsychological decline from childhood to midlifePNAS 2012 109 (40) E2657–E2664; published ahead of print August 27, 2012, doi:10.1073/pnas.1206820109 b) Elizabeth J. D'Amico, Joan S. Tucker, Jeremy N. V. Miles, Brett A. Ewing, Regina A. Shih, Eric R. Pedersen. Alcohol and Marijuana Use Trajectories in a Diverse Longitudinal Sample of Adolescents: Examining Use Patterns from Age 11to17. *Addiction*, 2016; DOI: 10.1111/add.13442

14. https://www.camh.ca/en/research/news_and_publications/reports_and_books/Documents/LRCUG.KT.PublicBrochure.15June2017.pdf

a) "Changing Demographics of Marijuana Initiation: Bad News or Good?", 107(6), pp. 833–834 American Journal of Public Health June 2017

15. https://www.canada.ca/en/healthcanada/news/2017/06/statement_from_theministerofhealthonthelower-riskcannabisuseguid.html

16. http://www.vancitybuzz.com/2015/04/64-people-hospital-vancouver-420/

17. http://www.cbc.ca/news/canada/british-columbia/vancouver-420-damage-at-sunset-beach-park-will-take-up-to-5-weeks-to-fix-1.4079331

18. http://www.denverpost.com/2017/05/20/denver-420-rally-ban/

19. Pew Research Centre April 14, 2015, Seth Motel

20. http://www.cannabisskunksense.co.uk/books-and-downloads/videos-detail/mental-health-marijuana-anti-marijuana-educational-video1

21. https://www.bing.com/videos/search?q=samhsa+may+3+2005+marijuana+press+-conference&qpvt=samhsa+may+3+2005+marijuana+press+conference&view=detail&mid=45BE250DC7E18A8EEAF045BE250DC7E18A8EEAF0&FORM=VRDGAR a) https://www.bing.com/videos/search?q=samhsa+may+3+2005+marijuana+press+conference&qpvt=samhsa+may+3+2005+marijuana+press+conference&view=detail&mid=4D198AF-141557E9004C54D198AF141557E9004C5&&FORM=VDRVRV

22. See 20

23. https://www.city-journal.org/html/don%E2%80%99t-legalize-drugs-11758.html

24. https://www.americamagazine.org/issue/100/myths-drug-legalization

25. http://www.cbsnews.com/news/how-morley-safer-convinced-americans-to-drink-more-wine/

26. http://www.medscape.com/viewarticle/824237

27. http://www.unicef.ca/en/press-release/new-unicef-report-poor-health-violence-alarming-rates-among-canadas-kids

28. Josiane Bourque, Mohammad H. Afzali, Maeve O'Leary-Barrett, Patricia Conrod. Cannabis use and psychotic-like experiences trajectories during early adolescence: the coevolution and potential mediators. *Journal of Child Psychology and Psychiatry*, 2017; DOI: 10.1111/jcpp.12765

29. http://montrealgazette.com/storyline/regular-marijuana-use-can-increase-psychosis-risk-in-teens-study

30. Osuch E. Marijuana Use in Youth from Bench to Bedside to Longitudinal Outlook. *Canadian Journal of Psychiatry Revue Canadienne de Psychiatrie.* 2016;61(6):316-317. doi:10.1177/0706743716644148. Permission Editor.

31. Lethal But Legal: Corporations, Consumption and Protecting Public Health, 2014, Nicholas Freudenberg, Distinquished Professor of Public Health, CUNY, USA a)http://www.tobaccoatlas.org/topic/tobacco-companies/

Notes

Chapter 1

1. www.focusonthefamily.com/socialissues/family/marijuana-the-big-picture/
where-theres-smoke-marijuana

2. See 1. Permission Rod Thomson June 16, 2017 www.therevoluntionaryact.com

3. Colorado Attorney General Cynthia Coffman, 2/2015. Verified by office of the Governor 6/21/2017.

4. The American Disease, Origins of Narcotic Control, David F. Musto, Oxford Press 1999

5. http://www.pbs.org/wgbh/pages/frontline/shows/dope/interviews/musto.html

6. Miech, R. A., Johnston, L. D., O'Malley, P. M., Bachman, J. G., & Schulenberg, J. E., & Patrick, M. E. (2017). *Monitoring the Future national survey results on drug use, 1975-2016:Volume I, secondary school students*. Ann Arbor: Institute for Social Research, The University of Michigan, Public Domain

7. Permission Mary Brett. www.cannabisskunksense.co.uk

8. http://www.cbc.ca/news/politics/pot-marijuana-legalization-consultations-1.3750985

9. http://www.ccsa.ca/Resource%20Library/CCSA-Medical-Use-of-Cannabis-Report-2016-en.pdf
Porath-Waller, A.J., Brown, J.E., Frigon, A.P., & Clark, H. (2013). What Canadian youth think about cannabis. Ottawa,ON: Canadian Centre on Substance Abuse.

10. http://www.cps.ca/en/documents/position/cannabis-children-and-youth

a) Boak A, Hamilton HA, Adlaf EM, Mann RE. Drug Use Among Ontario Students, 1977–2015: Detailed OSDUHS Findings. CAMH Research Document Series, No. 41. Toronto: Centre for Addiction and Mental Health, 2015

b) http://www.statcan.gc.ca/pub/85-002-x/2015001/article/14201-eng.htm- "60% of illicit drug users in Canada are between 15 and 24".

c) https://www.dosomething.org/us/facts/11-facts-about-teens-and-drug-use, see references

d) US data: https://www.nih.gov/news-events/news-releases/regular-marijuana-use-teens-continues-be-concern d) Substance Abuse & Mental Health Services Administration. "National Survey on Drug Use and Health: Summary of National Findings." Results from the 2012 National Survey on Drug Use and Health. Accessed February 25, 2014,e)http://www.samhsa.gov/data/NSDUH/2012SummNatFindDetTables/NationalFindings/NSDUHresults2012.htm.

11. https://www.drugabuse.gov/publications/principles-adolescent-substance-use-disorder-treatment-research-based-guide/frequently-asked-questions/it-possible-teens-to-become-addicted-to-marijuana

12. https://www.asam.org/docs/default-source/advocacy/marijuana-use-fact-sheet.pdf?sfvrsn=928a75c2_0#search="marijuana"

13. http://www.denverpost.com/2013/11/11/
pot-problems-in-colorado-schools-increase-with-legalization/

14. http://www.westword.com/news/
marijuana-colorado-education-association-opposing-amendment-64-5834662

a)http://reason.com/24-7/2012/09/19/colorado-teachers-union-opposes-marijuan

15. http://www.oregon.gov/oha/ph/PreventionWellness/marijuana/Documents/rmsac/rmsac-statements-adolescent-mj-use.pdf

16. https://hudson.org/research/11298-marijuana-and-school-failure Permission David Murray June 9, 2017

17. US Government, Federal Register, vol 54, no 249, 29 December 1989

18. G. Leighty, A. F. Fentiman Jr, and R. L. Foltz, Longretained metabolites of delta9- and delta8- tetrahydrocannabinols identified as novel fatty acid conjugates. Res Commun Chem Pathol Pharmacol 14, 13-28 (1976) a) http://www.able.org/studies/detox/drug_storage.pdf Public domain

19. http://www.consumerreports.org/content/dam/cro/news_articles/health/Consumer%20Reports_March-April_1975-Marijuana-Feature.pdf

20. https://www.researchgate.net/publication/300731294_The_Helsinki_Symposium_1975

21. https://www.canada.ca/en/health-canada/services/drugs-health-products/medical-use-marijuana/information-medical-practitioners/information-health-care-professionals-cannabis-marihuana-marijuana-cannabinoids.html

 a) http://www.dailymail.co.uk/news/article-4846328/Marijuana-makes-men-s-sperm-lazily-swim-circles.html

22. https://www.acog.org/Resources-And-Publications/Committee-Opinions/Committee-on-Obstetric-Practice/Marijuana-Use-During-Pregnancy-and-Lactation

23. http://www.abc.net.au/news/2012-07-18/study-finds-pregnancy-and-marijuana-a-dangerous-mix/4137666

24. https://www.researchgate.net/publication/21307384_Marijuana_carry-over_effects_on_aircraft_pilot_performance

 a) http://articles.orlandosentinel.com/1985-11-23/lifestyle/0340460232_1_ailerons-land-an-airplane-pilots

25. Study Finds Marijuana Affects Last 24 Hours, LA Times on December 1ˢᵗ, 1985, United Press International

26. https://archives.drugabuse.gov/NIDA_Notes/NNVol11N3/MarijMemory.html a) https://www.canada.ca/en/health-canada/services/substance-abuse/controlled-illegal-drugs/health-risks-of-marijuana-use.html

27. http://www.ccsa.ca/Resource%20Library/CCSA-Cost-of-Cannabis-Collisions-Canada-Infographic-2017-en.pdf a)http://www.sciencedirect.com/science/article/pii/S0376871617300686

28.http://cdpsdocs.state.co.us/ors/docs/reports/2016-SB13-283-Rpt.pdf

29.http://denver.cbslocal.com/2016/06/10/ban-on-pot-gummy-bears-signed-into-colorado-law/

30. https://learnaboutsam.org/wp-content/uploads/2017/02/06Feb2017-SAM-educational-briefs.pdf

31.http://mynews4.com/news/local/sparks-man-sentenced-to-40-years-in-prison-for-fatal-dui-crash-that-killed-two

32.https://www.si.com/racing/2014/09/24/tony-stewart-kevin-ward-racing-death-grand-jury

33.http://www.cbc.ca/news/canada/saskatchewan/coroner-report-released-death-regina-boy-haven-dubois-1.3390899 a)http://www.cbc.ca/news/canada/saskatchewan/marijuana-significant-factor-in-haven-dubois-death-1.3392179

Chapter 2

1. http://www.cbc.ca/news/canada/calgary/remedy-ice-cream-calgary-edible-marijuana-market-1.4056703

2. http://www.cbsnews.com/news/bloomberg-medical-marijuana-one-of-great-hoaxes-of-all-time/

3. Emory Wheel Newspaper February 6 1979

4. http://www.maps.org/news-letters/v04n2/04252lsd.html
The Summit Meeting Commemorating the 50th. Anniversary of the Discovery of LSD. April 1993

5. CNN May 9, 2009

6. http://jamanetwork.com/journals/jama/article-abstract/2338230

7. http://www.denverpost.com/2015/06/26/moment-of-truth-for-medical-marijuana/

8. Oregon Public Health Authority 2011

9. Colorado Department of Public Health and Environment 2011

10. https://gov.idaho.gov/mediacenter/Bills/S%201146.pdf Permission Governor's office

11. http://www.seattletimes.com/opinion/editorial-unregulated-medical-marijuana-market-is-creating-a-hazy-future/ Permission Seattle Times

12. http://www.thenewstribune.com/news/local/marijuana/article27459787.html

13. *On Marijuana*, 2015 Grafton and Scratch Publishers

14. http://healthycanadians.gc.ca/recall-alert-rappel-avis/hc-sc/2014/42677a-eng.php

15. http://ottawacitizen.com/news/local-news/
health-canada-warns-marijuana-producers-about-advertising

16. https://www.americanbar.org/content/dam/aba/administrative/healthlaw/health_mo_premium_hl_healthlawyer_v29_2802.authcheckdam.pdf

17. https://www.ncbi.nlm.nih.gov/pubmed/19596652

18. https://aidsinfo.nih.gov/news/12/fda-approves-new-indication-fordronabinol

19. https://www.asco.org/search/site/dronabinol?f[0]=fctSiteName%3AASCO.
org&f[1]=fctSiteName%3AMeeting%20Library

20. https://www.clinicalleader.com/doc/
insys-cbd-receives-orphan-status-from-fda-in-dravet-syndrome-0001

21. http://ir.gwpharm.com/releasedetail.cfm?ReleaseID=960348

22. http://www.duidvictimvoices.org/

Chapter 3

1. The Health Effects of Cannabis and Cannabinoids, National Academies of Sciences, Engineering and Medicine, USA 2017, Permission granted June 16, 2017 Josh Blatt

2. https://www.canada.ca/en/services/health/marijuana-cannabis/task-force-cannabis-legalization-regulation.html

3. Hall W. What has research over the past two decades revealed about the adverse health effects of recreational cannabis use? *Addiction*, 109: doi: 10.1111/add.12703

4. Lynskey M.T., Vink J.M., Boomsma D.I. Early onset cannabis use and progression to other drug use in a sample of Dutch twins. *Behav Genet* 2006;36:195-200

5. http://who.int/substance_abuse/publications/cannabis_report/en/index3.html Permission granted.

6. University of Bristol. "Teen cannabis use and illicit drug use in early adulthood linked: One in 5 adolescents at risk of tobacco dependency, harmful alcohol consumption and illicit drug use." Science Daily, 7 June 2017. <www.sciencedaily.com/releases/2017/06/170607222448.htm

7. https://www.drugabuse.gov/about-nida/noras-blog/2015/01/brain-in-progress-why-teens-cant-always-resist-temptation

8. Schoeler, T., Theobald, D., Pingault, J. B., Farrington, D. P., Jennings, W. G., Piquero, A. R., ... Bhattacharyya, S. (2016). Continuity of cannabis use and violent offending over the life course. *Psychological Medicine*, 1-15. DOI: 10.1017/S0033291715003001

9. https://www.stinson.com/Resources/Articles/2017_Articles/Emerging_Products_Liability_Threats_to_Growing_Marijuana_Industry.aspx

10. JAMA Psychiatry. (2016). Published online 31 August 2016. doi:10.1001/jamapsychiatry.2016.1728SIEC No: 20160446

11. http://www.addictionjournal.org/press-releases/what-twenty-years-of-research-on-cannabis-use-has-taught-us

a) http://www.foxnews.com/health/2014/10/07/marijuana-and-your-health-what-20-years-research-reveals.html

b) http://www.nydailynews.com/life-style/health/marijuana-mental-disorders-loss-intelligence-20-year-study-article-1.1965934

12. https://link.springer.com/article/10.1007/s10552-013-0259-0, Cancer Causes & Control October 2013, Volume 24, Issue 10, pp 1811–1820

13. American Chemical Society. "Marijuana Smoke Contains Higher Levels Of Certain Toxins Than Tobacco Smoke." *ScienceDaily*, 18 December 2007. www.sciencedaily.com/releases/2007/12/071217110328.htm

14. http://www.cfpc.ca/uploadedFiles/Resources/_PDFs/Authorizing%20Dried%20Cannabis%20for%20Chronic%20Pain%20or%20Anxiety.pdf Permission granted.

15. http://nationalpost.com/pmn/news-pmn/canada-news-pmn/new-brunswick-medical-society-launches-campaign-cautioning-against-marijuana-use/wcm/ddd31787-32da-4427-90c7-85b9ce0a1421

a) www.legalnotsafe.ca

16. http://www.cyanb.ca/images/NBOCYA_Submission_to_Select_Committee_on_Cannabis.pdf

Chapter 4

1. http://hitchensblog.mailonsunday.co.uk/2017/02/stupid-arguments-for-drug-legalisation-examined-and-refuted.html

2. Drug Free Australia

3. Drug Free Australia

4. http://www.unicef.org/malaysia/Drug_Abuse_and_its_impact_of_Children.pdf. Permission Unicef Malaysia

5. https://www.medicaljane.com/products/edibles/drinks/

6. https://www.stickyguide.com/dispensaries/kindpeoples-collective/products/hashman-cherry-bomb-wpot-rocks-bar

7. https://www.usnews.com/news/best-states/rhode-island/articles/2017-06-02/authorities-toddler-nearly-dies-from-edible-marijuana

Notes

8. Wilson KM, Torok MR, Wei B, et al. Marijuana exposure in children hospitalized for bronchiolitis. Available at: http://www. abstracts2view.com/pas/view.php? nu¼PAS16L1_4460.8. Accessed June 8, 2016.

9. https://familycouncil.org/?m=20170714

10. http://insider.foxnews.com/2017/01/11/
marijuana-edible-school-bus-massachusetts-boy-hospitalized

11. http://healthland.time.com/2013/05/28/
more-kids-accidentally-ingesting-marijuana-following-new-drug-policies/

12. https://www.statnews.com/2016/08/09/edible-marijuana-kids/

13. ABC News, September 5, 2014 Richmond, Virginia

14. https://www.centeronaddiction.org/about June 29, 2011 CNN

15. https://www.metlife.com/assets/cao/foundation/PATSFULL-ReportFINAL-May.pdf page 9

16. Monitoring Health Concerns Related To Marijuana In Colorado 2016. Colorado Department of Revenue

17. https://www.centeronaddiction.org/newsroom/press-releases/
casa-report-finds-more-teens-treatment-marijuana-alcohol-or-all-other

18. See 17

19. http://health.usnews.com/health-news/family-health/childrens-health/articles/2011/06/29/
addiction-starts-early-in-american-society-report-finds

20. A critique of cannabis legalization proposals in Canada, Kalant, Harold International Journal of Drug Policy, Volume 34, 5 - 10

21. https://www.tni.org/files/download/rise_and_decline_ch1.pdf

a) Mills (2003) Smoking hashish is still popular in Egypt and the harsh laws, including capital punishment, are rarely enforced. Page 160

22. Keep Off The Grass, Gabriel G. Nahas, M.D., Ph.D., D.Sc.1990

23. https://www.tni.org/en/publication/the-un-drug-control-conventions

24. https://treaties.un.org/Pages/ViewDetails.
aspx?src=TREATY&mtdsg_no=IV-11&chapter=4&lang=en

25. https://aifs.gov.au/cfca/publications/issues-safety-and-wellbeing-children-families/introduction

26. https://aifs.gov.au/cfca/publications/improving-outcomes-children-living-families-pare

27. https://www.gov.uk/government/uploads/system/uploads/attachment_data/file/120620/hidden-harm-full.pdf

28. https://archives.drugabuse.gov/about/welcome/aboutdrugabuse/magnitude/

29. https://www.acf.hhs.gov/cb

a) https://www.childwelfare.gov/pubPDFs/drugexposed.pdf

30. https://www.childwelfare.gov/pubPDFs/drugexposed.pdf

31. See 30

32. https://link.springer.com/article/10.1007/s10096-002-0699

a) http://www.cannabisskunksense.co.uk/articles/research-papers-detail/
fatal-aspergillosis-associated-with-smoking-contaminated-marijuana-in-a-mar

b) http://www.aspergillus.org.uk/content/marijuana-use-and-aspergillosis

33. https://www.canada.ca/en/health-canada/programs/consultation-toward-legalization-regulation-restriction-access-marijuana/discussion-paper-introduction.html

a)https://www.canada.ca/en/services/health/marijuana-cannabis/task-force-marijuana-legalization-regulation/framework-legalization-regulation-cannabis-in-canada.html

b) https://www.canada.ca/en/health-canada/programs/consultation-toward-legalization-regulation-restriction-access-marijuana/task-force-marijuana-legalization-regulation/summary-expertise-experience-affiliations-interests.html

34. http://docplayer.es/28931025-The-pontifical-academy-of-sciences-narcotics-problems-and-solutions-of-this-global-issue-november-2016-casina-pio-iv-vatican-city.html

35. http://www.unis.unvienna.org/unis/en/pressrels/2003/nar784.html

Chapter 5

1. Accessed December 12, 2016 http://www.whitehouse.gov/ondcp/marijuana

2. https://www.justice.gov/opa/pr/attorney-general-announces-formal-medical-marijuana-guidelines

3. https://www.justice.gov/opa/pr/justice-department-announces-update-marijuana-enforcement-policy

4. http://www.latimes.com/nation/la-na-medical-pot-20141216-story.html

5. https://learnaboutsam.org/sam-statement-regarding-removal-doj-marijuana-enforcement-barriers-proposed-cjs-appropriations-bill/

a) https://learnaboutsam.org/wp-content/uploads/2017/06/28Apr2017-SAM-Testimony-to-House-CJS-on-Medical-Marijuana-Language-final.pdf

b) http://thehill.com/homenews/senate/344204-senate-panel-advances-measure-to-protect-medical-marijuana-states

6. Letter April 23, 2015 Hon. Rona Ambrose

7. http://www.cbc.ca/news/politics/liberal-legal-marijuana-pot-1.4041902

8. http://www.ctvnews.ca/canada/too-early-to-gauge-pot-legalization-s-effect-on-criminal-market-rcmp-1.3362909

9. https://www.liberal.ca/realchange/marijuana/

a) http://www.cbc.ca/news/politics/philpott-un-marijuana-legislation-legalize-1.3544554

b) http://globalnews.ca/news/3544709/n-b-to-set-legal-marijuana-age-at-19-sale-through-crown-corporation/

10. https://www.nytimes.com/2017/04/13/world/canada/trudeau-marijuana.html?_r=0

11. http://mjinews.com/cannabis-canada-association-welcomes-government-canadas-proposed-cannabis-act/

12.Catherine Cullen tweet April 13, 2017

13. See 12

14. http://www.cbc.ca/news/politics/premiers-marijuana-legislation-1.4209113

15. https://openparliament.ca/politicians/alistair-macgregor/?page=6

Notes

16. https://petitions.ourcommons.ca/en/Petition/Details?Petition=e-1053

17. http://www.businessinsider.com/
spicer-says-justice-department-will-enforce-weed-laws-under-trump-2017-2

18. https://www.youtube.com/watch?v=jcTdXq0gvy8 a)
https://blumenauer.house.gov/media-center/press-releases/
congressman-earl-blumenauer-statement-white-house-press-sec-sean-spicer

19. http://www.politico.com/story/2017/02/federal-marijuana-enforcement-sean-spicer-235318

20. http://www.latimes.com/politics/essential/la-pol-ca-essential-politics-updates-lt-gov-newsom-
writes-president-trump-1487972853-htmlstory.html

21. See 20

22. http://www.pbs.org/newshour/rundown/watch-jeff-sessions-announc-
es-guidelines-stricter-sentencing/ a) https://www.washingtonpost.com/politics/
jeff-sessions-war-on-drugs-has-medical-marijuana-advocates-worried

23. https://www.justice.gov/opa/speech/
attorney-general-jeff-sessions-delivers-remarks-sergeants-benevolent-association-new-york

24. https://assets.documentcloud.org/documents/3913305/Sessions-Hickenlooper-July-24-2017-
Letter.pdf

25. Pediatric death/http://escholarship.org/uc/item/1n10w5pc#page-1

a) http://www.poppot.org/2017/09/07/pediatric-death-cannabis-exposure/

26. http://www.cpac.ca/en/programs/in-committee-house-of-commons/episodes/52691788

Chapter 6

1. http://druglibrary.net/schaffer/dea/pubs/cngrtest/ct961202.htm

2. https://www.followthemoney.org

3. http://www.drugpolicy.org/sites/default/files/Drug_Policy_Alliance-Financial%20
Statements_2012.pdf

a) https://projects.propublica.org/nonprofits/organizations/5215166

4. https://projects.propublica.org/nonprofits/organizations/521975211

5. https://www.forbes.com/sites/chloesorvino/2014/10/02/
an-inside-look-at-the-biggest-drug-reformer-in-the-country-george-soros/#42b315c71e29

6. https://www.dea.gov/docs/marijuana_position_2011.pdf*

a) http://www.realwomenofcanada.ca/the-un-meeting-on-drugs-reality/

b) http://www.cchrflorida.org/the-legalization-of-marijuana-part-1-of-2/

c) http://www.washingtontimes.com/news/2014/apr/2/
billionaire-george-soros-turns-cash-into-legalized/

7. http://nationalpost.com/news/canada/medical-mari-
juana-production-in-canada-set-for-dramatic-change/
wcm/76b93237-4deb-48ef-aa56-63f3dd81674f

8. Cannabis Inc., film documentary, reporter Ben Knight, Producer Suzanne Smith, Foreign
Correspondent ABC http://www.abc.net.au/foreign/content/2014/s4027079.htm

9. https://www.inc.com/will-yakowicz/cannabis-raised-104-million-venture-capital.html

a) https://www.cbinsights.com/research/cannabis-industry-market-map/

b) https://www.cbinsights.com/research/cannabis-startup-industry-funding/

10. http://fortune.com/2015/01/08/founders-fund-privateer-holdings/

11. https://www.rt.com/usa/206959-marley-family-weed-brand/

a) http://www.nbcnews.com/storyline/legal-pot/
stir-it-bob-marley-headline-corporate-cannabis-brand-n250286

b) http://www.itv.com/news/2014-11-18/bob-marley-to-be-face-of-the-first-global-pot-brand/

c) http://www.billboard.com/articles/business/6319944/bob-marley-natural-marijuana-brand

12. https://cannabisnow.com/new-york-times-runs-first-full-page-cannabis-ad/

a) http://www.telegraph.co.uk/finance/newsbysector/mediatechnologyandtelecoms/
media/11010764/New-York-Times-runs-full-page-marijuana-advert.html

b) https://www.fastcompany.com/3033929/
marijuana-startup-leafly-takes-out-full-page-ad-in-the-new-york-times

13. http://www.spokesman.com/stories/2015/apr/16/judge-doesnt-change-pot-rule/

a) http://www.poppot.org/2015/04/19/judge-upholds-the-schedule-i-classification/

b) https://casetext.com/case/united-states-v-pickard-22#!

14. https://casetext.com/case/united-states-v-pickard-22#!

15. https://www.washingtonpost.com/news/in-theory/wp/2016/04/29/5-reasons-marijua-
na-is-not-medicine/?utm_term=.e51baa831525

16. https://learnaboutsam.org/wp-content/uploads/2016/12/AMA_i13csaph2-summary-only.pdf

17. https://www.drugfree.org.au/images/pdf-files/library/Policies_Legislation_and_law/APA_
Position_Statement.pdf

18. https://static1.squarespace.com/static/5541a76ae4b0175cee8827d0/t/56e81d3bb-
654f9ada96a72c3/1458052412170/CBDlettertoPAv2.pdf

19. https://learnaboutsam.org/colorado-coalition-doctors-call-denver-post-leafly-stop-showcas-
ing-unfounded-medical-claims/

20. Permission Bob Doyle, Letter

21. www.leafly.com

22. See 21

23. http://www.csam-smca.org/wp-content/uploads/2013/09/CJA_Journal_September_2013.pdf

Chapter 7

1. https://object.cato.org/sites/cato.org/files/pubs/pdf/greenwald_whitepaper.pdf

2. http://content.time.com/time/health/article/0,8599,1893946,00.htm

3. http://www.cbc.ca/news/canada/toronto/erskine-smith-decriminalize-all-drugs-1.3958336

4. https://www.washingtonpost.com/opinions/five-myths-about-legalizing marijuana/2013/06/07/
9727eac4-c871-11e2-9f1a 1a7cdee20287_story.html? utm_term=.1d735217bc7d

5. https://learnaboutsam.org/five-errors-the-washington-post-shouldve-caught-about-marijuana/

Notes

6. MacCoun, R. & Reuter, P. (1997). Interpreting Dutch cannabis policy: Reasoning by analogy in the legalisation debate. Science, 278(3): 47–52; cf. de Zwart, W. & van Laar, M. (2001). Cannabis regimes. British Journal of Psychiatry, 178: 574 Evaluating alternative cannabis regimes a) ROBERT MacCOUN, PETER REUTER The British Journal of Psychiatry Feb 2001, 178 (2)123 128; DOI: 10.1192/bjp.178.2.123

a) http://bjp.rcpsych.org/content/178/2/123)http://research.omicsgroup.org/index.php/Drug_policy_of_the_Netherlands

b) http://www.emcdda.europa.eu/legal-topic-overviews/cannabis-possession-for-personal-use

c) https://www.researchgate.net/publication/7572454_Strong_increase_in_total_D9-THC_in_cannabis_preparations_sold_in_Dutch_coffee_shops

7. http://www.dutchnews.nl/news/archives/2016/12/amsterdams-oldest-cannabis-cafe-closes-because-of-school-rule/

8. Correspondence Smart Approaches to Marijuana Canada

9. http://www.druglibrary.org/crl/perspectives/Johnson%20&%20Gerstein%2098%20Usage%20Trends_%20AmJPubHealth.pdf

10. http://www.pbs.org/wgbh/pages/frontline/shows/drugs/cron/a)
http://archive.boston.com/bostonglobe/obituaries/articles/2010/10/15/dr_david_musto_authority_on_drug_control_policy_at_74/

11.http://www.nytimes.com/1986/11/17/us/anatomy-of-the-drug-issue-how-after-years-it-erupted.html

12. http://www.independent.co.uk/life-style/health-and-families/health-news/cannabis-an-apology-5332409.html

13. http://transform-drugs.blogspot.ca/2007/03/how-independent-on-sunday-got-it.html

a) http://anepigone.blogspot.ca/2007/03/harmful-consequences-of-marijuana-sees.html

14. https://www.independent.co.uk/voices/editorials/leading-article-the-cannabis-debate-5332542.html

15. https://www.gov.uk/government/uploads/system/uploads/attachment_data/file/98026/drug-strategy-2010.pdf

16.https://petition.parliament.uk/archived/petitions/104349

17. http://www.independent.co.uk/news/uk/politics/government-issues-damning-response-to-200000-signature-cannabis-legalisation-petition-10471713.html

a) See 16

18. EMCDDA http://www.ibtimes.co.uk/marijuana-legalisation-uk-falling-out-love-cannabis-1506697

19. Moore, THN, Zammit, S, Lingford-Hughes, A et al. Cannabis use and risk of psychotic or affective mental health outcomes: a systematic review. Lancet. 2007; 370: 319–328

a) Cannabis use and risk of psychotic or affective mental health outcomes: a systematic review Moore, Theresa HM et al. The Lancet, Volume 370, Issue 9584, 319 - 328

20.Correspondence with Pamela McColl and Dr. Philip Seeman

21, https://www.samhsa.gov/newsroom/press-announcements/201308220415

a) http://sam-vt.org/2016/01/25/marijuana-legalization-will-cost-taxpayers/

22.http://sam-vt.org/wp-content/uploads/2014/10/White-Paper-Press-Release.pdf

23. http://www.cannabisskunksense.co.uk/uploads/site-files/Cannabis_General_Facts_July_2015.pdf

24. https://www.eurekalert.org/pub_releases/2017-05/aaop-evr042617.php

25. Center for Behavioral Health Statistics and Quality. (2012). Treatment Episode Data Set (TEDS) 2000-2010: National admissions to substance abuse treatment services (DASIS Series S-61, HHS Publication No. SMA 12-4701). Rockville, MD: Substance Abuse and Mental Health Services Administration. Retrieved from http://www. samhsa.gov/data/2k12/TEDS2010N/TEDS2010NWeb.pdf

26. https://www.samhsa.gov/data/sites/default/files/CBHSQ128_1/CBHSQ128/sr128-typical-day-adolescents-2013.pdf

Chapter 8

1. http://tbac.us/2013/12/02/marijuana-cause-or-the-cure/

2. https://www.canada.ca/en/health-canada/services/drugs-health-products/medical-use-marijuana/licensed-producers/consumer-information-cannabis-marihuana-marijuana.html Permission granted Health Canada

3. Accessed on 7/28/16: http://www.thalidomide.ca/the-canadian-tragedy

4. http://www.thalidomide.ca/history-of-thalidomide/

5. Accessed on 8/4/16: http://www.contergan.grunenthal.info/grt-ctg/GRT-CTG/Die_Fakten/Chronologie/152700079.jsp

6. Accessed on 7/28/16: http://www.fda.gov/Drugs/NewsEvents/ucm320924.htm

7. Accessed on 7/29/16: http://news.gc.ca/web/article-en.do?nid=945369&tp=1

8. Reece AS, Hulse GK. Chromothripsis and epigenomics complete causality criteria for cannabis- and addiction-connected carcinogenicity, congenital toxicity and heritable genotoxicity. Mutat Res. 2016;789:15-25.

9. Accessed on 7/28/16: http://www.hc-sc.gc.ca/dhp-mps/marihuana/med/infoprof-eng.php

10. Accessed on 1/8/16: https://www.whitehouse.gov/ondcp/frequently-asked-questions-and-facts-about-marijuana#harmless

11. Accessed on 1/8/16: https://www.whitehouse.gov/ondcp/marijuana

12. http://nationalpost.com/news/toronto/ttc-wins-right-to-demand-random-drug-and-alcohol-tests-on-10000-drivers-other-workers/wcm/432a60b4-289a-41d3-aed9-50e71a8f595

13. Accessed on 7/28/16 http://www.fda.gov/drugs/drugsafety/postmarketdrugsafetyinformationforpatientsandproviders/ucm2008016.htm

14. Accessed on 7/28/16: https://www.revaid.ca/revaid/

Chapter 9

1. Asbridge M, Hayden JA, Cartwright JL. Acute cannabis consumption and motor vehicle collision risk: systematic review of observational studies and meta-analysis, BMJ 2012;344: e536.

   a. Laumon B, Gadegbeku B, Martin J-L, Biecheler M-B, SAM Group. Cannabis intoxication and fatal road crashes in France: population based case-control study. *BMJ* 2005;331:1371-7.

Notes

b. Drummer OH, Gerostamoulos J, Batziris H, et al. The involvement of drugs in drivers of motor vehicles killed in Australian road traffic crashes. *Accid Anal Prev* 2004;36:239-48.

c. Li M, Brady JE, DiMaggio CJ, et al. Marijuana use and motor vehicle crashes. *Epidemiol Rev* 2012;34:65-72.

d. Hartman R, Huestis M. Cannabis effects on driving skills. *Clin Chem* 2013;59:478-92.

2. Li G, Chihuri S, Brady JE. Role of alcohol and marijuana use in the initiation of fatal two-vehicle crashes. *Ann Epidemiol* 2017;27:342-347. (change "eight fold" to "six fold")

3. Code of Colorado Regulations, Marijuana enforcement Division, R 604 – Retail marijuana products manufacturing: health and safety regulations. Accessed 7/22/17

   a. Accessed 7/22/17. http://www.cnn.com/2016/10/21/health/colorado-marijuana-potency-above-national-average/

4. Monitoring Health Concerns Related to Marijuana in Colorado, 2016. Colorado Department of Public Health & Environment. Colorado.gov/cdphe/marijuana-health-report

5. Hartman RL, Brown TL, Milavetz G et al. Cannabis effects on driving lateral control with and without alcohol. *Drug Alcohol Depend* 2015;154:25-37.

6. Hartman RL, Richman JE, Hayes CE, Huestis MA. Drug Recognition Expert (DRE) examination characteristics of cannabis impairment. Accid Anal Prev 2016;92:219-29.

   a) http://www.rcmp-grc.gc.ca/ts-sr/aldr-id-cfa-aldr-eng.htm

7. DUID Victim Voices Tanya and Adrian Guevarra. Accessed on 7/22/17: http://www.duidvictimvoices.org/duid-victims/tanya-and-adrian-guevarra/

8. CBS/AP. Woman who plowed into Las Vegas crowd tested positive for marijuana. Accessed on 7/22/17: http://www.cbsnews.com/news/woman-lakeisha-holloway-who-plowed-car-into-las-vegas-crowd-tested-positive-for-marijuana/

9. Solomon R, Chamberlain E. Traffic Injury Prev. 2014; 15(7): 685-693.

10. Hedlund J. Drug-Impaired Driving: A guide for states. Governors Highway Safety Association. Foundation for Advancing alcohol responsibility. April 2017.

11. http://www.ccsa.ca/Resource%20Library/CCSA-Youth-Drugged-Driving-technical-report-2014-en.pdf

12. http://www.icadtsinternational.com/files/documents/2013_015.pdf

13. http://www.statcan.gc.ca/pub/85-002-x/2015001/article/14201-eng.htm

14. Salomonsen-Sautel S, Min SJ, Sakai JT, et al. Trends in fatal motor vehicle crashes before and after marijuana commercialization in Colorado. *Drug Alcohol Depend* 2014; 140:137-144.

   a) Grondel DT. Driver Toxicology Testing and the Involvement of Marijuana in Fatal Crashes, 2010-2014. A descriptive report. Washington Traffic Safety Commission. October 2015.

15. http://www.cbc.ca/news/canada/five-friends-killed-nine-injured-in-car-crash-1.189606

16. Permission to quote Richard Goodman, estate of Dr. Goodman,

17. DUID Victim Voices Rosemary Tempel. Accessed on 7/22/17: http://www.duidvictimvoices.org/duid-victims/rosemary-tempel/

18. Proposition 64 – California, Accessed on 7/22/17: http://vig.cdn.sos.ca.gov/2016/general/en/pdf/text-proposed-laws.pdf

19. Crancer A, Drum P. Medical marihuana involved in CA fatal crashes. 2014 Fatality Analysis Reporting System (FARS) NHTSA. February 2016. http://www-fars.nhtsa.dot.gov/Main/index.aspx

20. Crancer A, Drum P. Medical marijuana responsible for traffic fatalities. 2011 - 2015 Fatality Analysis Reporting System (FARS) NHTSA. September 2016. http://www-fars.nhtsa.dot.gov/Main/index.aspx

21. Governor's Highway Safety Association Drug-Impaired Driving A guide for what states can do, 2013 Fatality Analysis Reporting System (FARS). http://www.ghsa.org/resources/drug-impaired-driving-guide-what-states-can-do

22. Brady JE, Li G. Trends in alcohol and other drugs detected in fatally injured drivers in the United States, 1999-2010. *Am J Epidem* 2014.

23. Crancer A, Drum P. Medical marijuana responsible for traffic fatalities. 2011 - 2015 Fatality Analysis Reporting System (FARS) NHTSA. September 2016. http://www-fars.nhtsa.dot.gov/Main/index.aspx

24. Crancer A, Drum P. Medical marihuana involved in CA fatal crashes. 2014 Fatality Analysis Reporting System (FARS) NHTSA. February 2016. http://www-fars.nhtsa.dot.gov/Main/index.aspx

25. See 24

26. See 24

27. See 24

28. Crancer A, Drum P. Slow driving while marijuana impaired is a myth! 2014 Fatality Analysis Reporting System (FARS) NHTSA. April 2016. http://www-fars.nhtsa.dot.gov/Main/index.aspx

29. Hartman RL, Huestis MA. Cannabis effects on driving skills. *Clin Chem* 2013;59(3).

30. Crancer A, Drum P. Marijuana and DUI Fatal Crashes Differ by Time of Day and Day of Week. 2015 Fatality Analysis Reporting System (FARS) NHTSA. March 2017. http://www-fars.nhtsa.dot.gov/Main/index.aspx

31. Grondel DT. Driver toxicology testing and the involvement of marijuana in fatal crashes, 2010-2014 A descriptive report. Washington Traffic Safety Commission October 2015

32. Johnson G. More drivers positive for pot in Washington. Seattle Times March 2014. http://seattletimes.com/html/localnews/2023075967_apxmarijuanadrivingwashington.html

a) Crancer A, Drum P. Marijuana and DUI Fatal Crashes Differ by Time of Day and Day of Week. 2015 Fatality Analysis Reporting System (FARS) NHTSA. March 2017. http://www-fars.nhtsa.dot.gov/Main/index.aspx

33. http://health.costhelper.com/drug-alcohol-test.html

34. Wood E, Brooks-Russell A, Drum P. Delays in DUI blood testing: Impact on cannabis DUI assessments. *Traff Inj Prevent* 2016;17:2, 105-10.

35. Johnson G. More drivers positive for pot in Washington. Seattle Times March 2014. http://seattletimes.com/html/localnews/2023075967_apxmarijuanadrivingwashington.html

36. Ditzler G. Study: Percentage of THC impaired drivers jumped after marijuana legalization. Spokane News. September 2015. http://www.kxly.com/news/spokane-news/study-percentage-of-thc-impaired-drivers-jumped-after-marijuana-legalization/35210758

a) Grondel DT. Driver toxicology testing and the involvement of marijuana in fatal crashes, 2010-2014 A descriptive report. Washington Traffic Safety Commission October 2015

b) Accessed 10/11/15: http://wtsc.wa.gov/research-data/quarterly-target-zero-data/

37. National Highway Transportation Safety Administration, Fatality Analysis Reporting System (FARS), 2006-2013 and CDOT/RMHIDTA 2014

Notes

38. See 37

39. US Department of Transportation National Highway Traffic Safety Administration. *The Economic and Societal Impact Of Motor Vehicles Crashes, 2010 (revised) – accessed 9/30/15:* http://www-nrd.nhtsa.dot.gov/pubs/812013.pdf

40. Keyes S. Colorado's marijuana tax revenues nearly double last year's figures. September 2015. https://www.theguardian.com/us-news/2015/sep/21/colorado-marijuana-tax-revenues-2015

41. http://www.syracuse.com/crime/index.ssf/2015/06/father_given_visits_with_girl_4_after_smoking_pot_in_car_causing_near-fatal_cras.html#incart_m-rpt-1iving

42. http://rozeklaw.com/2016/03/05/man-admits-drug-alcohol-fatal-crash/

43. http://komonews.com/news/local/friends-family-hold-vigil-for-teens-killed-in-crash

44. https://issuu.com/pnwmarketplace/docs/i20150122230228989/3

45. https://www.multivu.com/players/English/8083051-state-farm-driving-marijuana/

46. http://www.cbc.ca/news/politics/cannabis-marijuana-legalization-driving-impaired-1.4191409

47. http://www.ccsa.ca/Resource%20Library/CCSA-Drug-Impaired-Driving-Toolkit-Facts-2016-en.pdf

48. http://vancouversun.com/news/local-news/trucking-industry-challenges-feds-on-marijuana-impaired-driving-standards

Chapter 10

1. http://www.rmhidta.org Vol.1 August 2013, The Legalization of Marijuana in Colorado

2. https://www.sciencedaily.com/releases/2013/05/130527231914.htm

3. George Sam Wang. Pediatric Marijuana Exposures in a Medical Marijuana StatePediatric Marijuana Exposures. *JAMA Pediatrics*, 2013; 1 DOI: 10.1001/jamapediatrics.2013.140

4. Salomonsen-Sautel, Stacy & T Sakai, Joseph & Thurstone, Christian & Corley, Robin & Hopfer, Christian. (2012). Medical Marijuana Use Among Adolescents in Substance Abuse Treatment. Journal of the American Academy of Child and Adolescent Psychiatry. 51. 694-702. 10.1016/j.jaac.2012.04.004.

5. http://www2.cde.state.co.us/artemis/hemonos/he1282m332015internet/he1282m332015internet01.pdf

6. kiro7news

7. kktvnews Black-market-marijuana-bust-leaves-bruises-on-Colorados-marijuana-industry

Chapter 11

1. http://www.ctvnews.ca/business/canopy-growth-says-number-of-medical-marijuana-patients-more-than-tripled-1.3284327

2. https://www.focusonthefamily.com/socialissues/citizen-magazine/marijuana/where-theres-smoke

3. https://www.livescience.com/53644-marijuana-is-stronger-now-than-20-years-ago.html

a) National Center for Natural Products Research (NCNPR), Research Institute of Pharmaceutical Sciences. Quarterly Report, Potency Monitoring Project, Report 107, September 16, 2009 thru December 15, 2009. University, MS: NCNPR, Research Institute of Pharmaceutical Sciences, School of Pharmacy, University of Mississippi (January 12, 2010).

b) Orens A, et al. Marijuana Equivalency in Portion and Dosage. An assessment of physical and pharmacokinetic relationships in marijuana production and consumption in Colorado. Prepared for the Colorado Department of Revenue. August 10, 2015.

4. https://www.asam.org/advocacy/find-a-policy-statement/view-policy-statement/public-policy-statements/2012/07/30/white-paper-on-state-level-proposals-to-legalize-marijuana

5. Wagner, F.A. & Anthony, J.C. (2002). From first drug use to drug dependence; developmental periods of risk for dependence upon marijuana, cocaine, and alcohol. *Neuropsychopharmacology* 26, 479-488.

a) Budney, A. J., Vandrey, R. G., Hughes, J. R., Thostenson, J. D., & Bursac, Z. (2008). Comparison of cannabis and tobacco withdrawal: Severity and contribution to relapse. *Journal of Substance Abuse Treatment, 35*(4), 362-368.

6. Dr. Eric Voth, Institute on Global Drug Policy a) http://tbac.us/wp-content/uploads/2013/01/MARIJUANA-THE-HARMS-HANDOUT-010513.pdf

7. http://www.theolympian.com/news/local/marijuana/article54985485.html

a) http://www.poppot.org/2016/03/09/psychosis-is-increasing/

8. https://parenting.blogs.nytimes.com/2014/02/10/that-six-serving-bar-of-marijuana-chocolate-my-son-ate-it/?_r=0

9. http://www.cbsnews.com/news/two-denver-deaths-tied-to-recreational-marijuana-use/

10. https://www.csmonitor.com/USA/Latest-News-Wires/2014/0403/Pot-cookie-blamed-in-falling-death-of-Colorado-student

11. http://www.cbsnews.com/news/man-fatally-shoots-himself-after-eating-5-marijuana-candies/

12. http://docplayer.net/17188193-Annual-update-barbara-brohl-executive-director-colorado-department-of-revenue-ron-kammerzell-deputy-senior-director-of-enforcement.html Annual Update: Colorado Department of Revenue 2015.

13. See 12

14. //www.colorado.gov/pacific/sites/default/files/PF_Youth_MJ-Infographic-Digital.pdf

15. https://www.forbes.com/sites/elizabethlopatto/2014/04/24/marijuana-legalization-what-about-the-teens/#542e18d43932

16. https://niaaa.nih.gov/news-events/news-releases/prevalence-marijuana-use-among-us-adults-doubles-over-past-decade

17. https://www.readbyqxmd.com/read/25841223/cannabis-withdrawal-a-new-diagnostic-category-in-dsm-5 https://www.drugabuse.gov/sites/default/files/parents_mj_brochure_2016.pdf

18. See 17

19. http://datia.org/datia/resources/latestopcannabis.pdf

20. http://www.businesswire.com/news/home/20091103005128/en/AllTranz-Awarded-4-Million-Research-Grant-NIH a)http://drugdelivery.pharmaceutical-business-review.com/news/alltranz_receives_4m_research_grant_from_nih_nida_091103

21. http://www.bendbulletin.com/opinion/2514404-151/letter-vote-no-on-marijuana-legalization-to-save

a) http://thechart.blogs.cnn.com/2014/04/16/casual-marijuana-use-may-damage-your-brain/

b) Cannabis Use Is Quantitatively Associated with Nucleus Accumbens and Amygdala Abnormalities in Young Adult Recreational Users

Notes

22. Jodi M. Gilman, John K. Kuster, Sang Lee, Myung Joo Lee, Byoung Woo Kim, Nikos Ma kris, Andre van der Kouwe, Anne J. Blood, Hans C. Breiter Journal of Neuroscience 16 April 2014, 34 (16) 5529-5538; DOI:10.1523/JNEUROSCI.4745-13.2014

23. See 22, 24

24. Hall and Degenhardt 2009

25. Christine Miller, Ph.D.

26. https://www.canada.ca/en/services/health/marijuana-cannabis/task-force-cannabis-legaliza-tion-regulation.html

27. Peter Hitchens

28. Christine Miller, Ph.D.

29. Chttp://www.justice.gc.ca/eng/rp-pr/other-autre/c45

30. https://www.ptsd.va.gov/professional/co-occurring/marijuana_use_ptsd_veterans.asp

31. See 30

32. Christine Miller, PhD.

33. Cannabis use disorder and suicide attempts in Iraq/Afghanistan-era veterans. Kimbrel, Nathan A. et al.Journal of Psychiatric Research,Volume 89 , 1 - 5

34.The National Academies of Sciences, Engineering, and Medicine, Health and Medicine Division, Board on Population Health and Public Health Practice, Committee on the Health Effects of Marijuana: An Evidence Review and Research Agenda. The Health Effects of Cannabis and Cannabinoids: The Current State of Evidence and Recommendations for Research. Washington, DC, January 12, 2017 http://nationalacademies.org/hmd/Reports/2017/health-ef-fects-of-cannabis-and-cannabinoids.aspx

35. http://www.psychiatrist.com/jcp/article/Pages/2015/v76n09/v76n0925.aspx

36. http://www.nhregister.com/colleges/article/Yale-study-raises-concern-over-medical-marijuana-11342320.php

    a) http://www.medscape.com/viewarticle/836588

37. http://www.psychiatrist.com/jcp/article/Pages/2015/v76n09/v76n0925.aspx

38. https://www.mentalhealth.va.gov/docs/2016suicidedatareport.pdf

    a) https://www.uspharmacist.com/article/suicide-in-the-veteran-population

39. https://learnaboutsam.org/new-study-finds-marijuana-abuse-linked-suicide-attempts-iraqaf-ghanistan-era-veterans/

40. http://www.cbc.ca/news/canada/nova-scotia/marijuana-treatment-for-ptsd-unproven-says-veterans-affairs-minister-erin-o-toole-1.3073007

41. See 40

42. http://www.ctvnews.ca/politics/auditor-urges-veterans-affairs-to-rein-in-medical-marijuana-use-costs-1.2885280

43. http://www.cbc.ca/news/politics/veterans-hehr-pot-policy-1.3861534

44. http://www.veterans.gc.ca/eng/about-us/reports/departmental-audit-evaluation/2016-review-marijuana-medical-purposes/summary

45. https://www.tilray.ca/en/news/ubc-and-tilray-launch-canadas-first-clinical-trial-to-study-medical-cannabis-and-ptsd/

a) https://tworowtimes.com/news/regional/
canadas-first-clinical-trial-study-medical-cannabis-ptsd/

46. http://janinafisher.com/pdfs/addictions.pdf Jane Fisher, Ph.D., November 13, 2000 Addiction and Trauma Recovery

47. Drug Alcohol Depend. 2015 Nov 1;156:70-77. doi: 10.1016/j.drugalcdep.2015.08.036. Epub 2015 Sep 25.

Chapter 12

1.Miech, R. A., Johnston, L. D., O'Malley, P. M., Bachman, J. G., & Schulenberg, J. E. (2015). Monitoring the Future national survey results on drug use, 1975–2014: Volume I, Secondary school students. Ann Arbor: Institute for Social Research, The University of Michigan. Available at http://monitoringthefuture.org/pubs.html#monograp hs

2. Substance Abuse and Mental Health Services Administration, *Results from the 2010 National Survey on Drug Use and Health: Summary of National Findings*, NSDUH Series H-41, HHS Publication No. (SMA) 11-4658. Rockville, MD: Substance Abuse and Mental Health Services Administration, 2011.

3. https://www.centeronaddiction.org/newsroom/press-releases/
national-study-reveals-teen-substance-use-america%E2%80%99s-1-public-health-problem

4. https://learnaboutsam.org/national-survey-shows-colorado-still-1-state-country-marijuana-use-18-25-year-old-use-rate-skyrocketing/

5. http://www.rmhidta.org/html/FINAL%20Denver%20Post%20HKCS%20Response%20(3).pdf

6. https://www.rand.org/news/press/2010/07/07.html

7. http://www.businessinsider.com/marijuanas-getting-cheaper-in-colorado-2016-9

8. http://www.who.int/substance_abuse/publications/cannabis_report/en/index4.html

9. Marsha Schuchard, The Family Versus The Drug Culture, 1978.

10. Correspondence Smart Approaches to Marijuana Canada

11. Correspondence Smart Approaches to Marijuana Canada

12. "It Takes Longer, but When It Hits You It Hits You!": Videos About Marijuana Edibles on YouTube Melissa J. Krauss, Shaina J. Sowles, Haley E. Stelzer-Monahan, Tatiana Bierut & Patricia A. Cavazos-Rehg Substance Use & Misuse Vol. 52 , Iss. 6,2017

Chapter 13

1. https://dalgarnoinstitute.org.au/images/resources/pdf/cannabis-conundrum/Tracking_
Marijuana_Money.pdf

2. Followthemoney.org

3. http://samaction.net/wp-content/uploads/2016/05/SDDA-Analysis_AUMAAct_Final.pdf

4. http://www.shouselaw.com/concentrated-cannabis
http://www.poppot.org/2017/01/24/butane-hash-oil-fires-grow-legalization/

5. October 26, 2016 http://www.cbsnews.com/
news/60-minutes-colorado-governor-on-recreational-pot/

6. https://www.unodc.org/documents/ungass2016/Contributions/Civil/DrugFreeAustralia/DFAs_
Position_on_Medical_Marijuan_2014.pdf

7. Pike G, Medical Marijuana, May, 2013

Notes

Chapter 14

1. http://www.richmond.com/opinion/their-opinion/guest-columnists/rafael-lemaitre-column-the-next-big-tobacco-makes-inroads-into/article_ea41f4cc-96ee-55f6-8b45-32cb27e7f223.html

2. https://ohsonline.com/Articles/2014/09/01/Marijuana-Legalization.aspx?Page=1

3. https://www.cdc.gov/pcd/issues/2014/13_0293.htm

4. http://globalnews.ca/news/2651785/
nova-scotia-political-leaders-lukewarm-on-pot-as-legalization-looms/

5. http://www.canadianbusiness.com/business-news/
legal-marijuana-sales-boost-tax-collections-but-the-drug-no-budget-cure-all/

   a) http://globaldrugpolicy.org/Issues/Vol%207%20Issue%204/Vol7Issue4sm.pdf

6. http://azdhs.gov/documents/licensing/medical-marijuana/reports/2016/mm fy16-year-end-report.pdf
http://azdhs.gov/licensing/medical-marijuana/index.php June 2017 Pregnancy

7. http://www.santacruzsentinel.com/article/zz/20130306/NEWS/130308010

8. https://oag.ca.gov/system/files/initiatives/pdfs/15-0069%20%28Medical%20Marijuana%29.pdf

9. http://www.washingtontimes.com/news/2015/jan/14/
george-soros-funds-ferguson-protests-hopes-to-spur/

10. Monitoring Health Concerns Related to Colorado, 2016 Colorado Department of Revenue

11. https://www.fairwarning.org/2017/02/rjreynoldssharptonmentholrestrictions/

12. https://afro.com/legalizing-weed-not-answer/

13. http://tobaccocontrol.bmj.com/content/14/3/172

14. US Secretary of Health, Education and Welfare 1979

15. USA Today May 31, 2011

16. https://www.nytimes.com/2014/11/02/education/edlife/this-is-your-brain-on-drugs-marijuana-adults-teens.html?_r=0

17. Persistent cannabis users show neuropsychological decline from childhood to midlife PNAS 2012 109 (40) E2657–E2664; 2012, doi:10.1073/pnas.1206820109

18. https://www.theguardian.com/world/2017/apr/10/canada-marijuana-industry-new-brunswick

19. See 18.

   a) Child Rights Impact Assessment New Brunswick http://www.cyanb.ca/images/NBOCYA_Submission_to_Select_Committee_on_Cannabis.pdf b)http://www.cbc.ca/news/canada/new-brunswick/organigram-marijuana-retail-new-brunswick-1.4291255

20. http://www.businessinsider.com/jobs-marijuana-legalization-industry-2014-7

21. http://www.cbc.ca/news/canada/ottawa/
smiths-falls-celebrates-tweed-s-medical-marijuana-licence-1.2515893

22. http://www.npr.org/sections/theprotojournalist/2014/05/08/310707885/13-spliffy-jobs-in-the-marijuana-industry

23. https://www.cbsnews.com/news/60-minutes-five-states-to-vote-on-recreational-pot/

24. http://www.huffingtonpost.ca/entry/jerry-brown-marijuana_n_4885455

25. PNAS Plus - Social Sciences - Psychological and Cognitive Sciences:Persistent cannabis users show neuropsychological decline from childhood to midlifePNAS 2012 109 (40) E2657–E2664; published ahead of print August 27, 2012, doi:10.1073/pnas.1206820109

26. http://www.gloucestertimes.com/opinion/column-state-making-a-mistake-on-marijuana/article_74ac4e03-82ee-513f-86ef-348badf6e27c.ht

27. http://www.cbc.ca/news/canada/north/
pilot-s-pot-use-a-factor-in-n-w-t-fatal-plane-crash-1.1329354

28. US Department of Transportation

29. http://www.privateerholdings.com/blogmaster/2015/11/17/
leafly-places-nations-first-cannabis-company-advertisement-in-the-new-york-times-print-edition

30. http://www.sfchronicle.com/nation/article/Judge-gives-her-reasons-for-deciding-that-pot-is-6207859.php

31. https://www.washingtonpost.com/news/in-theory/wp/2016/04/29/5-reasons-marijuana-is-not-medicine/?utm_term=.ae29f10b8304

Chapter 15

1. http://www.drugpolicy.org/drug-facts/10-facts-about-marijuana/marijuana-medicinal-properties

2. Cannabis Inc. Foreign Correspondent ABC News Australia

3. http://www.macleans.ca/news/canada/why-its-time-to-legalize-marijuana/

4. http://www.drugpolicy.org/mission-and-vision

5. http://www.camh.ca/en/hospital/about_camh/influencing_public_policy/Documents/
CAMHCannabisPolicyFramework.pdf

   a) Room et al., 2010: 72

6. https://www.bjs.gov/content/pub/pdf/p09.pdf

   a) https://learnaboutsam.org/the-issues/marijuana-and-whos-in-prison

7. http://drthurstone.com/times-lapse-in-judgment/

8. https://townhall.com/columnists/rachelalexander/2015/08/03/
no-one-serves-jail-time-for-smoking-pot-n2033738

9. https://www.bjs.gov/content/dcf/enforce.cfm

   a) https://www.prisonpolicy.org/scans/whos_in_prison_for_marij.pdf

10. http://gazette.com/legalization-didnt-unclog-prisons/article/1548308

11. Communication with Smart Approaches to Marijuana Canada a) https://www.researchgate.net/
publication/277890794_The_Nature_and_Extent_of_Marihuana_Possession_in_British_Columbia

12. https://www.bjs.gov/content/dcf/duc.cfm

13. The Role of Marijuana in Homicide Barry Spunt, Paul Goldstein, Henry Brownstein & Michael Fendrich International Journal of the Addictions Vol. 29 , Iss. 2,1994

14. http://drthurstone.com/times-lapse-in-judgment/

15. https://www.change.org/p/no-marijuana-grows-in-snohomish-county-r5-zones-no-recreational-marijuana-stores-in-clearview-maltby-lake-stevens-hwy-9-corridor-limit-medical-marijuana-to-1-mile-do-not-grandfather-in-existing-medical-marijuana-shops

Notes

16. https://globalnews.ca/news/1526890/
marijuana-ticketing-option-in-the-hands-of-government-police-chiefs/

17. http://www.cbc.ca/news/politics/
marijuana-reform-5-things-to-know-about-possible-changes-to-the-law-1.2560834

18. https://whataboutweed.org/archives/3020

19. http://www.ncpa.org/pub/bg148?pg=5

a) https://www.government.nl/topics/youth-crime/reducing-youth-crime

20. http://www.mensjournal.com/travel/articles/
inside-the-marijuana showdown-at-the-canadian-border-w483596

21. http://www.macleans.ca/news/canada/
if-youve-ever-smoked-marijuana-beware-of-the-u-s-border/

22. http://thefederalist.com/2015/11/24/
legalized-marijuana-just-smoked-my-sons-job-prospects-through-the-roof/

23. http://www.sciencedirect.com/science/article/pii/S0955395916301529

24. http://www.camh.ca/en/hospital/about_camh/influencing_public_policy/Documents/
CAMHCannabisPolicyFramework.pdf

25. Juvenile Law Center

26. http://time.com/4298038/marijuana-history-in-america/

27. https://www.usnews.com/education/blogs/student-loan-ranger/2015/04/15/
drug-convictions-can-send-financial-aid-up-in-smoke

28. The American Disease, Dr. David Musto

29. http://www.cedro-uva.org/lib/harrison.cannabis.03.html

30. https://www.nytimes.com/topic/subject/rockefeller-drug-laws

31. https://www.youtube.com/watch?v=uCvdvpY0LWg

32. http://content.time.com/time/nation/article/0,8599,1888864,00.html

33. https://bjs.gov/content/pub/pdf/Felsent.pdf

34. Cannabis Use in the United States Implications for Policy.

35. http://www.nytimes.com/1994/02/12/opinion/ms-reno-and-the-jail-glut.html

a) See 29

36. https://townhall.com/columnists/rachelalexander/2015/08/03/
no-one-serves-jail-time-for-smoking-pot-n2033738

Chapter 16

1. Gazette Editorial Board July 8, 2016 http://gazette.com/editorial-big-marijuana-trashes-democratic-process/article/1579890 Permission to Reprint on Behalf of the Editor/Dan Steever April 5,2017

2. https://ballotpedia.org/Ohio_Marijuana_Legalization_Initiative,_Issue_3_(2015)

3. Tracking the Money That's Legalizing Marijuana And Why It Matters Sue Rusche President and CEO National Families in Action

4. http://www.rmhidta.org/html/FINAL%20NSDUH%20Results-%20Jan%202016%20Release.pdf

5. http://www.cbsnews.com/news/
teenagers-perception-marijuana-changing-as-more-states-legalize-pot/

6. Has Legal Pot For Adults Impacted Teens' Use of Drugs Dangers, *CBS* January 3, 2017

7. https://learnaboutsam.org/new-data-shows-colorado-youth-marijuana-use-rise-since-legalization/

8. https://www.hudson.org/research/12615-misrepresenting-colorado-marijuana
http://www.cannabisskunksense.co.uk/articles/press-article/letter-to-governor-hickenlooper"

9. Correlates of intentions to use cannabis among US high school seniors in the case of cannabis legalization Palamar, Joseph J. et al. *International Journal of Drug Policy*, Volume 25 , Issue 3 , 424-435

10. http://www.denverpost.com/2016/12/23/drug-child-welfare-cases-colorado-have-in-creased-in-colorado-but-connection-to-legalized-marijuana-is unclear/

a)http://america.aljazeera.com/articles/2015/9/7/parents-face-child-abuse-investiga-tions-over-marijuana-use.html#

11. http://www.cbsnews.com/news/60-minutes-five-states-to-vote-on-recreational-pot/

12. https://www.colorado.gov/pacific/sites/default/files/Market%20Size%20and%20Demand%20Study,%20July%209,%202014%5b1%5d.pdf
Market Size and Demand for Marijuana in Colorado (v16) Colorado Department of Revenue.

13. http://www.poppot.org/category/featured-2/news-articles/

Chapter 17

1. http://denver.cbslocal.com/2015/05/18/marijuana-intoxication-blamed-in-more-deaths-inju-ries/a) http://www.poppot.org/2017/09/15/enough-enough-n/

2. http://www.healthvermont.gov/stats/surveys

3. Thomas H. A community survey of adverse effects of cannabis use. Drug Alcohol Depend. 1996 Nov;42(3):201-7. Smith MJ, Thirthalli J, Abdallah AB, Murray RM, Cottler LB.

a)Prevalence of psychotic symptoms in substance users: a comparison across substances. Compr Psychiatry. 2009 May-Jun;50(3):245-50. Barkus EJ, Stirling J, Hopkins RS, Lewis S. Psychopathology. Cannabis-induced psychosis-like experiences are associated with high schizotypy 2006;39(4):175

b)http://www.othersideofcannabis.com/uploads/9/5/1/5/9515724/marijuanamythscm.pdf

4. http://onlinelibrary.wiley.com/doi/10.1111/ajad.12529/pdf

5. http://www.sfgate.com/politics/article/Momentum-to-legalize-marijuana-in-California-is-5880897.php

6. http://www.herkimercountyprevention.org/Marijuana.pdf

a) http://www.huffingtonpost.ca/entry/medical-marijuana-study-w_n_907521

7. http://www.huffingtonpost.com/sue-rusche/marijuana-legalization-pr_b_2884765.html

a)http://www.drugpolicy.org/drug-facts/10-facts-about-marijuana/marijuana-cancer

8. www.vice.com/en_uk The Pot Industry is a long way from being successful.

9. CBC News The National (2015) Wendy Mesley interview with John Moore

10. http://www.ibtimes.co.uk/marijuana-legalisation-uk-falling-out-love-cannabis-1506697

11. https://www.biosciencetechnology.com/news/2014/04/
marijuana-use-may-result-heart-related-complications-young-middle-aged-adults

Notes

12. Association between cannabis use and methadone maintenance treatment outcomes: an investigation into sex differences Biology of Sex Differences, 2017, Volume 8, Number 1, Page 1 Laura Zielinski, Meha Bhatt, Nitika Sanger, *Biology of Sex Differences*2017**8**:8 https://doi.org/10.1186/s13293-017-0130-1 Creative Commons Attribution 4.0 International License (http://creativecommons.org/licenses/by/4.0/), (http://creativecommons.org/publicdomain/zero/1.0/)

13. http://www.canorml.org/healthfacts/healthmyths.html

   a) Medill Report – Natalie Pacini

   b) http://azdhs.gov/licensing/medical-marijuana/index.php

   c) http://azdhs.gov/documents/licensing/medical-marijuana/dispensaries/marijuana-warning-pregnancy.pdf

14. Survey of medicinal cannabis use among childbearing women; Patterns of its use in pregnancy and retroactive self-assessment of its efficacy against 'morning sickness' Complementary Therapies in Clinical Practice, Volume 15, Issue 4, November 2009, Pages 242-246

   a)June 2007 issue of Heads Magazine

15. http://ccsa.ca/Resource%20Library/CCSA-Cannabis-Maternal-Use-Pregnancy-Report-2015-en.pdf

   a) https://www.drugabuse.gov/publications/research-reports/marijuana/what-scope-marijuana-use-in-united-states

16. Substance Abuse and Mental Health Services Administration [SAMHSA], 2013)

17. http://ccsa.ca/Resource%20Library/CCSA-Cannabis-Maternal-Use-Pregnancy-Report-2015-en.pdf

   a) SAMHSA 2013

18. https://www.ncbi.nlm.nih.gov/pmc/articles/PMC3638200/

19. http://ccsa.ca/Resource%20Library/CCSA-Cannabis-Maternal-Use-Pregnancy-Report-2015-en.pdf

20. Monitoring Changes In Marijuana Use Patterns 2017, Colorado Department of Revenue 2017

21. http://jamanetwork.com/journals/jama/fullarticle/2594398

22. Marijuana Myths, Marijuana Facts, Drs. John. M. Morgan, Lynn Zimmer 1996

23. 'Prince of Pot' website recommends marijuana for pregnant women, Ada Slivinski, QMI Agency April 10, 2015

24. http://americanpregnancy.org/pregnancy-health/illegal-drugs-during-pregnancy/

25. http://ronaldlkirkish.blogspot.ca/2014/08/marijuana-and-pregnancy-what-are-risks.html

26. Giedd, J.N. (2004). Structural magnetic resonance imaging of the adolescent brain. Annals of the New York Academy of Sciences. 1021, 77-85.

   a) Hall, W. & Degenhard, L. (2009). Adverse health effects of non-medical cannabis use. Lancet. 374, 1383-1391.

   b) Tetrault, J.M. (2007). Effects of cannabis smoking on pulmonary function and respiratory complications: a systematic review. Archives of Internal Medicine. 167, 221-228.

   c) Hoffman, D., Brunnemann, K.D., Gori, G.B. & Wynder, E.E.L. (1975). On the carcinogenicity of marijuana smoke. In: V.C. Runeckles, Ed., Recent Advances in Phytochemistry. New York: Plenum.

d) Moore, T.H., Zammit, S., Lingford-Hughes, A. et al., (2007). Cannabis use and risk of psychotic or affective mental health outcomes: A systematic review. Lancet. 370 (9584), 319-328.

e) Large, M., Sharma, S., Compton, M., Slade, T. & Nielssen, O. (2011). Cannabis use and earlier onset of psychosis: a systematic meta-analysis. Archives of General Psychiatry. 68(6), 555-561.

f) Arseneault, L., Cannon, M, Poulton, R., Murray, R., Caspi, A., & Moffitt, T.E. (2002). Cannabis use in adolescence and risk for adult psychosis: longitudinal prospective study. British Medical Journal. 325, 1212-1213.

g) Wagner, F.A., & Anthony, J.C. (2002). From first drug use to drug dependence; developmental periods of risk for dependence upon cannabis, cocaine, and alcohol. Neuropsychopharmacology. 26, 479-488.

h) Fried, P.A. (1982). Marihuana use by pregnant women and effects on offspring: an update. Neurotoxicology and Teratology. 4, 451-454.

i) Goldschmidt, L., Day, N.L., Richardson, G.A. (2000). Effects of prenatal marijuana exposure on child behavior problems at age 10. Neurotoxicology and Teratology. 22, 325-336.

j) Jaddoe, V.W.V., van Duijn, C.M., Franco, O.H., van der Heijden, A.J. et al., (2012). The Generation R Study: design and cohort update 2012. European Journal of Epidemiology. 27, 739-756.

k) Fried, P.A. Watkinson, B. (2000). Visuoperceptual functioning differs in 9-12 year olds prenatally exposed to cigarettes and marijuana. Neurotoxicology and Teratology 22, 11-20.

l) Richardson, G.A., Ryan, C., Willford, J et al., (2002). Prenatal alcohol and marijuana exposure: effects on neuropsychological outcomes at 10 years. Neurotoxicology and Teratology. 24, 309-320.

m) Smith, A.M., Fried, P., Hogan, M., Cameron, I. (2006). Effects of prenatal marijuana on visuospatial working memory: An fMRI study in young adults. Neurotoxicology and Teratology. 28, 286-295.

n) Smith, A.M., Fried, P., Hogan, M., Cameron, I. (2004). Effects of prenatal marijuana exposure on response inhibition: An fMRI study of young adults. Neurotoxicology and Teratology. 26(4), 533-542.

o) Fried, P.A. & Smith, A. (2001). A literature review of the consequences of prenatal marihuana exposure: an emerging theme of a deficiency in aspects of executive function. Neurotoxicology and Teratology. 23, 1-11.

27. http://www.cclt.ca/Eng/topics/Treatment-and-Supports/Substance-Use-during-Pregnancy/Pages/default.aspx

28. http://www.cclt.ca/Eng/topics/Treatment-and-Supports/Substance-Use-during-Pregnancy/Pages/default.aspx

29. http://www.marchofdimes.org/pregnancy/marijuana.aspx

30. http://whoopiandmaya.com/find-whoopi-maya-products/

31. http://www.mamabirth.com/2012/10/smoking-marijuana-while-breastfeeding.html

32. Garry, A., Rigourd, V., Amirouche, A., Fauroux, V., Aubry, S., & Serreau, R. (2009). Cannabis and Breastfeeding. Journal of Toxicology, 2009, 596149. http://doi.org/10.1155/2009/596149

33. J Neuroendocrinol. 2008 May;20 Suppl 1:75-81. doi: 10.1111/j.1365-2826.2008.01670.x. Multiple roles for the endocannabinoid system during the earliest stages of life: pre- and postnatal development.

34. http://www.thedenverchannel.com/news/local-news/study-looking-at-effects-of-marijuana-use-on-breast-milk

Notes

35. http://www.denverpost.com/2016/05/01/
pueblo-hospitals-doctors-worried-about-new-mothers-marijuana-use/

36. Motherwisk.com

37. http://www.motherisk.org/women/updatesDetail.jsp?content_id=347

38. http://www.independent.co.uk/news/world/americas/cannabis-tampons-foria-relief-peri-od-painkiller-cramps-lower-back-pain-a7220381.html

39. Cannabis Inc. Documentary Film, Suzanne Smith Producer, Foreign Correspondent ABC Australia

40. See 39

41. https://www.nytimes.com/2014/11/02/education/edlife/this-is-your-brain-on-drugs-marijuana-adults-teens.html?_r=0

42. Should You Worry About Marijuana Edibles In Your Kid's Hallowe'en Treats? October 30, 2014, www.thequardian.com

43. https://ncnorml.com/why-this-matters/

44. Accessed on 8/1/2016:
https://www.drugabuse.gov/news-events/nida-notes/2010/12/marijuana-linked-testicular-cancer
Lacson JCA, et al. Population-based case-control study of recreational drug use and testis cancer risk confirms an association between marijuana use and nonseminoma risk. *Cancer.* 2012;118(21):5374-5383.Daling JR, et al. Association of marijuana use and the incidence of testicular germ cell tumors. *Cancer.* 2009;115(6):1215-1223.Gurney J, et al. Cannabis exposure and risk of testicular cancer: a systematic review and meta-analysis. *BMC Cancer* 2015;15:1-10.

45. http://www.cannabisskunksense.co.uk/articles/press-article/
kathy-gyngell-did-cannabis-trigger-the-westminster-killers-madness

   a) Simona A. Stilo,MD; Robin M. Murray RM. Translational Research 2010: The epidemiology of schizophrenia: replacing dogma with knowledge. Dialogues Clin Neurosci. 2010 Sep;12(3):305–315

46. http://denver.cbslocal.com/2015/05/18/
marijuana-intoxication-blamed-in-more-deaths-injuries/

   a) http://denver.cbslocal.com/2014/04/24/
edibles-the-main-culprit-when-it-comes-to-marijuana-hospital-visits/

47. https://www.brit-thoracic.org.uk/document-library/news/press-releases-2014-wm/
press-release-cannabis-emphysema-final-2014/

48. https://medicalxpress.com/news/2014-12-uk-verge-steep-lung-disease.html

49. Jodi M. Gilman, John K. Kuster, Sang Lee, Myung Joo Lee, Byoung Woo Kim, Nikos Makris, Andre Van Der Kouwe, Anne J. Blood and Hans C. Breiter. Cannabis Use is Quantitatively Associated with Nucleus Accumbens and Amygdala Abnormalities in Young Adult Recreational Users. *Journal of Neuroscience*, April 16, 2014

   a) Society for Neuroscience (SfN). "Brain changes associated with casual marijuana use in young adults, study finds." ScienceDaily. ScienceDaily, 15 April 2014. <www.sciencedaily.com/releases/2014/04/140415181156.htm

   b)https://www.nytimes.com/2014/11/02/education/edlife/this-is-your-brain-on-drugs-marijuana-adults-teens.html

50 https://d3r5by4xdsowev.cloudfront.net/Tracking_the_Money_Thats_Legalizing_Marijuana_and_Why_It_Matters_FINAL-R_3.15.2017-R.pdf

51. https://www.eurekalert.org/pub_releases/2013-05/uocd-sic052413.php

52. https://www.childrenscolorado.org/about/news/2014/march-2014/marijuana-safe-packaging-bill/

53. Half-Baked — The Retail Promotion of Marijuana Edibles Robert J. MacCoun, Ph.D., and Michelle M. Mello, J.D., Ph.D. N Engl J Med 2015; 372:989-991March 12, 2015DOI: 10.1056/NEJMp1416014

54. http://www.sacbee.com/opinion/california-forum/article172977841.html

Chapter 18

1. https://www.usnews.com/news/business/articles/2015/07/13/marijuana-opponents-using-racketeering-law-to-fight-industry

2. See 1

3. See 2

4. http://www.pbs.org/wgbh/pages/frontline/shows/settlement/interviews/blakey.html

5. http://www.ibtimes.com/holiday-inn-marijuana-lawsuit-against-colorado-pot-group-calls-nationwide-boycott-1823130

6. http://www.ibtimes.com/holiday-inn-marijuana-lawsuit-against-colorado-pot-group-calls-nationwide-boycott-1823130

7. http://www.cbsnews.com/news/hershey-wins-trademark-lawsuit-against-colorado-pot-company/

8. https://www.wsj.com/articles/lab-rat-ads-warn-teens-of-pot-use-1412560470

9. http://www.denverpost.com/2014/08/09/colorado-ad-campaign-tests-new-message-to-prevent-teen-marijuana-use/

10. http://drugfreecalifornia.org/PDF/CDFCCaliforniaListing10.pdf

11. http://www.newsmax.com/TheWire/san-jose-marijuana-ban/2016/11/02/id/756701/

12. http://www.westernfreepress.com/2015/07/16/arizona-voters-oppose-marijuana-legalization-initiative/

13.http://sfappeal.com/2013/05/california-supreme-court-rules-that-cities-and-counties-can-ban-medical-marijuana-dispensaries/

Oregon bans https://www.leafly.com/news/politics/oregon-cities-ban-cannabis

14. https://www.colorado.gov/pacific/sites/default/files/2014%20MED%20Annual%20Report_1.pdf

   a) http://www.lorainadas.org/wp-content/uploads/the-colorado-truth.pdf

Chapter 19

1. Alaska Marijuana Legalization, Ballot Measure 2 (2014) - Ballotpedia

2. Alaska Marijuana Legalization, Ballot Measure 2 (2014) - Ballotpedia

3. http://mjinews.com/alaska-marijuana-control-board-releases-full-regulations/

4. https://d3r5by4xdsowev.cloudfront.net/Tracking_the_Money_Thats_Legalizing_Marijuana_and_Why_It_Matters_FINAL-R_3.15.2017-R.pdf

5. http://www.orlandosentinel.com/news/politics/political-pulse/os-john-morgan-medical-marijuana-lawsuit-20170706-story.html

Notes

6. https://ballotpedia.org/Florida_Right_to_Medical_Marijuana_Initiative,_Amendment_2_(2014)

a) http://www.oregonlive.com/marijuana/index.ssf/2017/08/big_profits_extra_pot_fuel_ill.html

7. https://www.forumresearch.com/forms/News%20Archives/News%20Releases/50140_Federal_Trudeau_-_Marijuana_%2824082013%29_Forum_Research.pdf

8. https://www.camh.ca/en/hospital/about_camh/influencing_public_policy/Documents/CAMHCannabisPolicyFramework.pdf

9. http://legalite.ca/legal-news/laws/poll-canadas-marijuana-laws/

10. http://globalnews.ca/news/2173919/majority-of-canadians-support-decriminalizing-marijuana-poll/ a) http://nationalpost.com/news/canada/more-than-two-thirds-of-canadians-want-marijuana-laws-softened-though-a-majority-still-against-legalization-poll

11. A critique of cannabis legalization proposals in Canada
Kalant, Harold International Journal of Drug Policy , Volume 34 , 5 - 10

12. http://www.mainstreetresearch.ca/trudeau-narrowly-wins-debate/

13. https://rvoh.net/kids-marijuana-and-mad-men/

14. http://nationalpost.com/opinion/jeff-jedras-liberals-get-help-from-pro-pot-group/wcm/f3d9a4ae-9130-4ad5-8d30-b187af8929c9

15. Gallop.com

16. Gallop.com

17. https://www.bostonglobe.com/metro/2017/07/08/mass-towns-balking-pot-shops-beacon-hill-weighs-tighter-local-approvals/XXfCK4ERMhTvbI5PFBWsNK/story.html

18. http://www.businessinsider.com/roadblocks-to-marijuana-advertising-2014-4

19. http://www.ccohs.ca/oshanswers/legisl/billc45.html

20. http://business.financialpost.com/investing/marijuana-stocks-lose-ground-as-new-federal-government-legislation-remains-hazy-on-details

21. http://www.huffingtonpost.ca/entry/pot-smoking-santa_n_6348692

22. https://www.ncadd.org/blogs/in-the-news/new-data-shows-colorado-youth-marijuana-use-on-the-rise-since-legalization

23. The Cigarette Century, The Rise, Fall, and Deadly Persistence of the Product That Defined America, Allan M. Brandt 2007

24. https://www.ncadd.org/about-addiction/signs-and-symptoms/what-to-look-for-signs-and-symptoms.

a) Colorado kids http://www.rmhidta.org/html/FINAL%20Denver%20Post%HKCS%20Response%20(3).pdf

Chapter 20

1. http://gfarmalabs.com/index.html

2. http://10cigarettes.com/camel-cigarettes-an-advertising-trick/

3. https://www.cdc.gov/tobacco/data_statistics/fact_sheets/tobacco_industry/marketing/index.htm

4. https://www.tobaccofreekids.org/

5. http://global.tobaccofreekids.org/files/pdfs/en/APS_youth_set_en.pdf
https://www.cdc.gov/tobacco/data_statistics/fact_sheets/tobacco_industry/marketing/index.htm

6. http://ftcalliance.com/wp-content/uploads/2014/03/Tobacco-Industry-Denormalization-Booklet.pdf

7. http://www.tobaccoatlas.org/topic/tobacco-companies/

8. https://www.thestreet.com/story/12951851/1/altrias-untapped-40-billion-market-marijuana-in-the-us.html

9. http://www.who.int/tobacco/surveillance/survey/gats/en/

10. http://www.tobaccoatlas.org/topic/cigarette-use-globally/

11. https://www.tobaccofreekids.org/facts_issues

12. https://www.cdc.gov/mmwr/preview/mmwrhtml/ss5704a1.htm

a) Tried to quit https://www.canada.ca/en/health-canada/services/canadian-tobacco-alcohol-drugs-survey/2013-supplementary-tables.html

13. Cannabis Inc. http://www.abc.net.au/foreign/content/2014/s4027079.htm

14. https://www.bloomberg.com/news/articles/2017-04-06/pot-companies-flock-to-canada-as-u-s-laws-stymie-share-listings?cmpid%3D=socialflow-twitter-canada

15 http://www.latimes.com/business/la-fi-pot-legalization-20140603-story.html

16. https://www.milbank.org/wp-content/files/documents/featured-articles/pdf/Milbank_Quarterly_Vol-92_No-2_2014_The_Tobacco_Industry_and_Marijuana_Legalization.pdf

17. http://washingtonmonthly.com/2012/10/31/the-tobacco-industrys-longstanding-desire-to-sell-marijuana-cigarettes/ a) https://learnaboutsam.org/marijuana-is-like-tobacco/

a) http://www.npr.org/2014/10/30/360217001/kennedy-are-we-ready-for-big-tobacco-style-marketing-for-marijuana

18. http://www.newsmax.com/finance/Companies/Tobacco-Companies-Moving-Pot/2014/06/03/id/574988/

19. https://www.thestreet.com/story/12951851/2/altrias-untapped-40-billion-market-marijuana-in-the-us.html

20. https://www.milbank.org/quarterly/articles/waiting-for-the-opportune-moment-the-tobacco-industry-and-marijuana-legalization/

21. http://www.businessinsider.com/legal-marijuana-set-to-outsell-cereal-2017-3

22. http://www.businessinsider.com/legal-marijuana-set-to-outsell-cereal-2017-3

23. http://www.huffingtonpost.ca/entry/marijuana-industry-fastest-growing_n_6540166

24. https://www.arcviewmarketresearch.com/media-coverage

25. http://www.investopedia.com/news/legal-marijuana-federal-level-2021-arcview/

26. https://www.forbes.com/forbes/welcome/?toURL=https://www.forbes.com/sites/forbestreptalks/2016/06/14/this-facebook-alums-gum-startup-is-chewing-off-a-piece-of-cas-2-7b-medical-cannabis-market/&refURL=https://www.bing.com/&referrer=https://www.bing.com/

27. http://www.livescience.com/23562-secondhand-smoke-kills-nonsmokders.html

28. http://www.who.int/mediacentre/factsheets/fs339/en/

29. https://www.cdc.gov/tobacco/data_statistics/fact_sheets/fast_facts/index.htm

30. http://newsroom.heart.org/news/secondhand-marijuana-smoke-may-damage-blood-vessels-as-much-as-tobacco-smoke

31. Matthew Springer, Ph.D See 30

Notes

32. https://www.eurekalert.org/pub_releases/2015-05/jhm-et051215.php

   a) http://www.hopkinsmedicine.org/news/media/releases/
extreme_exposure_to_secondhand_cannabis_smoke_causes_mild_intoxication

33. https://oehha.ca.gov/media/downloads/proposition-65/chemicals/finalmjsmokehid.pdf

34. See 33

35. https://assets.bouldercounty.org/wpcontent/uploads/2017/04/Monitoring_Health_Concerns_
Report_FINAL.pdf

36. https://www.aap.org/en-us/about-the-aap/aap-press-room/pages/Colorado-Study-Finds-One-
in-Six-Children-Hospitalized-for-Lung-Inflammation-Positive-for-Marijuana-Exposure.as

37. See 36

Chapter 21

1. http://www.jti.com/media/news-releases/
jti-acquires-ploom-intellectual-property-rights-ploom-inc/

   a) https://www.questia.com/newspaper/1P2-38021089/
pot-smoking-without-the-smoke-marijuana-vapor-pens

2. https://www.nytimes.com/2015/01/13/health/with-the-e-joint-the-smoke-clears-.html

3. https://www.cdc.gov/media/releases/2013/p0905-ecigarette-use.html

4. http://www.tobaccofreekids.org/tobacco_unfiltered/tag/e-cigarettes

5. https://www.cdc.gov/media/releases/2013/p0905-ecigarette-use.html

6. See 5

7. http://www.dailynews.com/health/20150128/
why-california-declared-vaping-e-cigarettes-a-public-health-threat

8. https://www.cdc.gov/media/releases/2015/p0416-e-cigarette-use.html

9. http://www.monitoringthefuture.org/

10. http://www.prnewswire.com/news-releases/poisoning-calls-about-e-cigarettes-and-liquid-nico-
tine-more-than-doubled-in-2014--fda-must-act-to-protect-kids-300019

11. http://abcnews.go.com/Health/childs-death-liquid-nicotine-reported-vaping-gains-popularity/
story?id=27563788

12. https://tobacco.ucsf.edu/california-health-groups-strongly-support-cdph-educational-cam-
paign-e-cigarettes

   a) https://tobacco.ucsf.edu/analysis-smoking-ordinances-and-electronic-ciga-
rettes-which-used-oppose-including-ecigs-clean-indoor-air-laws

13. http://realfarmacy.com/study-reveals-e-cigarettes-toxic/

14. https://drugfree.org/learn/drug-and-alcohol-news/e-cigarette-vapor-can-contain-high-concen-
trations-formaldehyde-study/

   a) http://tobaccofreeca.com/secondhand-smoke/
new-tobacco-control-laws-effective-june-92016/

15. http://www.nejm.org/doi/full/10.1056/NEJMc1413069#t=article

16. https://www.cdc.gov/media/releases/2017/p0320-ecigarettes.html

17. http://www.newyorker.com/magazine/2014/12/08/natural-4

18. http://www.timesheraldonline.com/article/NH/20150718/SPORTS/150719862

19. http://www.cbsnews.com/news/e-cigarettes-dont-help-smokers-quit-study/

20. https://www.bloomberg.com/news/articles/2016-03-24/marlboro-kicks-some-ash

21. http://blogs.findlaw.com/free_enterprise/2014/05/candy-snack-companies-want-names-off-e-cigs.html

22. http://blog.center4tobaccopolicy.org/cease-and-desist-letters-sent-to-e-cigarette-companies/

23. http://ca.complex.com/pop-culture/2014/05/brands-issue-cease-and-desist-letters-to-e-cigarette-makers

24. http://www.cbc.ca/news/health/e-cigarette-liquid-nicotine-makers-fight-to-keep-candy-flavour-names-1.2654233

25. http://blogs.findlaw.com/free_enterprise/2014/05/candy-snack-companies-want-names-off-e-cigs.html

26. http://www.poppot.org/2017/03/13/girl-scouts-sue-marijuana-industry-get-results/

27. http://www.poppot.org/2017/03/13/girl-scouts-sue-marijuana-industry-get-results/

28. https://www.pinterest.com/pin/519180663272155869/?lp=true

29. https://weedmaps.com/strains/platinum-girl-scout-cookies-3

Chapter 22

1. http://tobaccocontrol.bmj.com/content/21/2/87.full

a) http://onlinelibrary.wiley.com/doi/10.1046/j.1440-1843.2003.00483.x/full

2. http://www.bmj.com/content/321/7257/323

3. https://www.cdc.gov/mmwr/preview/mmwrhtml/mm4843bx.htm

4. http://archive.tobacco.org/Documents/dd/ddfrankstatement.html

5. http://archive.tobacco.org/News/98minnesota.html

6. http://news.minnesota.publicradio.org/features/199805/08_stawickie_history/

7. http://www.abajournal.com/magazine/article/july_12_1957_surgeon_general_links_smoking_and_lung_cancer/stay_connected/newsletter

8. https://www.cancer.org/latest-news/the-study-that-helped-spur-the-us-stop-smoking-movement.html

9. http://ash.org.uk/information-and-resources/briefings/key-dates-in-the-history-of-anti-tobacco-campaigning/

10. https://www.rcplondon.ac.uk/projects/outputs/smoking-and-health-1962

11. https://profiles.nlm.nih.gov/ps/retrieve/Narrative/NN/p-nid/60

12. http://www.nejm.org/doi/pdf/10.1056/NEJMsa1211127

a) N Engl J Med 2013;368:351-64. DOI: 10.1056/NEJMsa1211127

13. http://www.nejm.org/doi/full/10.1056/NEJMe1213751 New Evidence That Cigarette Smoking Remains the Most Important Health Hazard Steven A. Schroeder, M.D.N Engl J Med 2013; 368:389-390January 24, 2013DOI: 10.1056/NEJMe1213751

Notes

14. Pierce JP, Choi WS, Gilpin EA, Farkas AJ, Berry CC. Tobacco industry promotion of cigarettes and adolescent smoking. JAMA. 1998;279(7):511-5. [CrossRef] [PubMed] a) https://www.ftc.gov/news-events/press-releases/1999/07/ftcs-annual-report-congress-cigarette-sales-and-advertising-1997

15. https://www.surgeongeneral.gov/library/reports/50-years-of-progress/sgr50-chap-5.pdf

   a) http://www.nytimes.com/1988/05/17/us/surgeon-general-asserts-smoking-is-an-addiction.html

16. http://www.publichealthlawcenter.org/sites/default/files/resources/master-settlement-agreement.pdf a)http://dictionary.sensagent.com/Tobacco%20Master%20Settlement%20Agreement/en-en/

17. https://www1.tobaccofreekids.org/index.php

   a) https://www.tobaccofreekids.org/research/factsheets/pdf/0156.pdf

18. https://www.scribd.com/document/94495669/Trends-in-Tobacco-Industry-Marketing

   a) U.S. Federal Trade Commission (FTC), Cigarette Report for 2003, 2005 [data for top six manufacturers only] http://www.ftc.gov/reports/cigarette05/050809cigrpt.pdf. FTC, Federal Trade Commission Smokeless Tobacco Report for the Years 2000 and 2001, August 2003, http://www.ftc.gov/os/2003/08/2k2k1smokeless.pdf [top five manufacturers].

19. http://globaltobaccocontrol.org/sites/default/files/lectures/en/pdf/tobaccoControl-2.1b.pdf

20. See 18

21. http://archive.sph.harvard.edu/press-releases/2007-releases/press01182007.html

   a) http://academic.laverne.edu/~ear/te/TEMain/News/NewsNicotineRise.htm

22. https://digital.library.unt.edu/ark:/67531/metacrs891/m1/1/high_res_d/RL30058_1999Nov05.html a) http://www.tobaccofreedom.org/issues/trends/prices/index.html

23. https://www.theguardian.com/society/2015/mar/12/plain-packaging-to-thank-for-australias-decline-in-smoking-says-labor

24. http://cigarettestime.com/cigarettes-articles/davidoff-id-cigarettes-by-imperial-tobacco

25. https://www.forbes.com/forbes/welcome/?toURL=https://www.forbes.com/sites/katiasavchuk/2015/03/18/michael-bloomberg-and-bill-gates-launch-4-million-legal-fund-to-fight-tobacco-industry/&refURL=https://www.bing.com/&referrer=https://www.bing.com/

   a) https://www.bloomberg.org/press/releases/bloomberg-philanthropies-bill-melinda-gates-foundation-launch-anti-tobacco-trade-litigation-fund/

26. http://www.prnewswire.com/news-releases/tobacco-carve-out-in-tpp-major-victory-for-public-health-300154193.html

27. http://www.justiceontobaccofraud.ca/

28. http://www.publichealthlawcenter.org/sites/default/files/resources/Tobacco-Control-Legal-Consortium-Cigarette-Graphic-Warnings-and-the-Divided-Federal-Courts.pdf

29. http://www.reuters.com/article/us-usa-cigarettes-labels-idUSBRE87N0NL20120824

30. https://www.canada.ca/en/services/health/marijuana-cannabis/task-force-marijuana-legalization-regulation/framework-legalization-regulation-cannabis-in-canada.html

31. https://www.theguardian.com/business/2015/dec/15/imperial-tobacco-drop-tobacco-from-name

   a)https://www.fool.com/investing/2017/06/16/cigarette-giant-imperial-brands-marijuana.aspx

   c) https://www.reuters.com/article/us-imperial-tobacco-namechange/imperial-tobacco-plans-to-change-name-to-imperial-brands-idUSKBN0TY1W220151215

32. http://www.independent.co.uk/news/business/comment/as-imperial-tobacco-hires-a-medical-marijuana-expert-can-legalised-dope-save-the-industry-a7789566.htm

Chapter 23

1. http://www.psaresearch.com/success4.html

2. D. E. Apollonio, R. E. Malone; Turning negative into positive: public health mass media campaigns and negative advertising. *Health Educ Res* 2009; 24 (3): 483-495. doi: 10.1093/her/cyn046

3. https://www.thetruth.com/

4. http://nbatc.ca/en/uploads/TID_GarMahood_PDF_001.pdf

   a) http://nsra-adnf.ca/wp-content/uploads/2016/08/TID_Booklet.pdf

5. See 4

6. See 4

7. http://hc-sc.gc.ca/hc-ps/pubs/tobac-tabac/ns-sn/index-eng.php

8. http://www.ohchr.org/Documents/Publications/GuidingPrinciplesBusinessHR_EN.pdf

9. https://www.unfairtobacco.org/en/pressrelease-quitpmi/

10. https://www.pmi.com/who-we-are/designing-a-smoke-free-future

11. University of Bath. "Number Of Russian Women Smokers Has Doubled Since Soviet Collapse." ScienceDaily, 29 January 2008. <www.sciencedaily.com/releases/2008/01/080128113304.htm>.

12. 2009, Global Adult Tobacco Survey

13. Lunze and Migliorini: Tobacco control in the Russian Federation- a policy analysis. BMC Public Health 2013 13:64.

14. See 11

15. http://www.huffingtonpost.com/2012/10/09/mitt-romney-bain-tobacco_n_1949812.html

16. Allen M. Brandt, *The Cigarette Century*

17. Letter copied to Smart Approaches to Marijuana Canada

18. Letter copied to Smart Approaches to Marijuana Canada

19. http://www.abc.net.au/foreign/content/2014/s4027079.htm
Cannabis Inc. Documentary Film 2014. Foreign Correspondent – Suzanne Smith Producer

20. http://www.timescolonist.com/news/b-c/prescription-pot-producer-plans-cross-country-tour-1.2259759

21. http://www.cbc.ca/news/business/tilray-export-marijuana-1.3628554

22. https://ca.finance.yahoo.com/news/tilray-announces-medical-cannabis-export-130000074.html

23. https://www.tilray.ca/en/news/tilray-exports-medical-cannabis-extracts-to-chile/

   a) https://qz.com/1080156/legalize-weed-lesotho-malawi-and-south-africa-are-all-closer-to-africas-first-legal-marijuana-license/

24. https://www.theglobeandmail.com/report-on-business/canopy-growth-posts-wider-loss-sees-patient-base-double/article35474499/

Notes

25. https://www.canada.ca/en/health-canada/programs/future-tobacco-control/future-tobac-co-control.html

26. The National Institute on Drug Abuse Blog Team. Brain and Addiction. Retrieved from https://teens.drugabuse.gov/drug-facts/brain-and-addiction on July 27, 2017.

27. https://www.omicsonline.org/references/marijuana-and-tobacco-a-major-connec-tion-1234497.html

Chapter 24

1. http://whyquit.com/NRT/WSJ_Helliker_Nicotine_Fix_020807.html

2. Chapman S, MacKenzie R (2010) The Global Research Neglect of Unassisted Smoking Cessation: Causes and Consequences. PLoS Med 7(2): e1000216. https://doi.org/10.1371/journal.pmed.1000216 Permission Open Access

3. https://www.nicorette.com.au/products

4. https://www.hsph.harvard.edu/news/press-releases/nicotine-replacement-therapies/ Permission Marge Dwyer/Harvard School of Public Health

5. Fiore MC, Bailey WC, Cohen SJ, et al. Treating Tobacco Use and Dependence. Clinical Practice Guideline. Rockville, MD: U.S. Department of Health and Human Services. Public Health Service. June 2000 page 4

6. http://bcrt.ca/premier-christy-clark-announces-free-support-to-help-smokers/

7. https://harmreductionjournal.biomedcentral.com/articles/10.1186/1477-7517-3-37

8. Baby and Me – Tobacco Free, Adam L., McColl P.

9. http://www.oregonlive.com/marijuana/index.ssf/2014/10/blue_dream_proves_popular_mari.html

10. http://www.reuters.com/article/us-pmi-who-fctc-tobacco-exclusive-idUSKBN19Y1DN

11. http://www.dailymail.co.uk/health/article-4950206/Smoking-cannabis-DOES-make-people-violent.html

12. Persistency of cannabis Use Predicts Violence following acute Psychiatric Discharge Jules R. Dugré1,2, Laura Dellazizzo1,2, Charles-Édouard Giguère1 , Stéphane Potvin1,2* and Alexandre Dumais Centre de recherche de l'Institut Universitaire en Santé Mentale de Montréal, Montréal, QC, Canada, Department of Psychiatry, Faculty of Medicine, Université de Montréal, Montreal, QC, Canada, 3 Institut Philippe-Pinel de Montréal, Montréal, QC, Canada

Chapter 25

1. http://nationalpost.com/news/canada/after-200-years-santa-kicks-a-bad-hab-it-publisher-activist-update-twas-the-night-before-christmas-take-away-st-nicks-pipe/wcm/6a93ffae-99a7-4ac0-94f2-6f9feb2041fe

2. NPR interview with Pamela McColl 2012.

3. http://www.cbc.ca/thecurrent/popupaudio.html?clipIds=2316189650 December 14, 2012 10:50

4. Correspondence with Grafton and Scratch, May 13, 2013

5. http://www.dailymail.co.uk/news/article-2222815/Publisher-axes-Santas-smoking-pipe-edits-classic-Night-Before-Christmas-poem-book-prompts-cries-censorship.html

6. http://www.ctvnews.ca/canada/
santa-goes-smoke-free-in-b-c-woman-s-rewriting-of-twas-the-night-before-christmas-1.10749

7. http://www.philstar.com/lifestyle-features/2012/12/12/885209/santa-kicks-smoking-habit

8. https://www.theguardian.com/books/2012/oct/24/santa-pipe-new-night-before-christmas

9. https://www.gov.uk/government/news/
all-children-really-want-this-christmas-is-their-parents-to-quit-smoking

10. Hassunah, R. and McIntosh, J. (2016) Quality of Life and Cannabis Use: Results from Canadian Sample Survey Data. *Health*,8,1576-1588. doi: 10.4236/health.2016.814155.

11. http://www.cbc.ca/news/canada/montreal/
the-reasons-behind-quebec-s-surprising-pessimism-toward-legalizing-pot-1.4133375

12. 3/4/2017, Lander, Wyoming KTVQ.com; Marijuana contributed to Wyoming triple fatal crash.

Notes Accessed as of October 4, 2017

For updates and links to current research, news stories and important developments on marijuana drug policy follow The Pied Pipers of Pot on facebook.